EBURY
THE 4-G CODE TO

Ishi Khosla is a practising clinical nutritionist, consultant, columnist, researcher, writer and entrepreneur. She is actively involved in clinical practice at the Centre for Dietary Counselling in Delhi, where she deals with a wide range of food and nutrition-related health problems. She started her career with the All India Institute of Medical Sciences, and later she was the head of the Nutrition Department of Preventive Cardiology at the Escorts Heart Institute and Research Centre, New Delhi, for several years. Passionate about nutrition, she spearheaded a health food company, Whole Foods India, which is in the business of producing and retailing health foods and operating health cafés. Ishi Khosla founded the Celiac Society of India in 2006 to spread awareness about celiac disease, a condition caused by wheat intolerance.

ALSO BY THE SAME AUTHOR

Is Wheat Killing You?
The Diet Doctor

THE 4-G
CODE to GOOD HEALTH

Don't Diet, *Know* What's Right for Your Body

ISHI KHOSLA

EBURY
PRESS

An imprint of Penguin Random House

EBURY PRESS

USA | Canada | UK | Ireland | Australia
New Zealand | India | South Africa | China

Ebury Press is part of the Penguin Random House group of companies
whose addresses can be found at global.penguinrandomhouse.com

Published by Penguin Random House India Pvt. Ltd
4th Floor, Capital Tower 1, MG Road,
Gurugram 122 002, Haryana, India

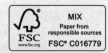

Penguin
Random House
India

First published in Ebury Press by Penguin Random House India 2022

ISBN 9780143453031

Typeset in Sabon by MAP Systems, Bengaluru, India
Printed at Replika Press Pvt. Ltd, India

www.penguin.co.in

Contents

PART II: What Should We Do?

Introduction

Dear Reader,

We all know that we live in the information age. Books, magazines, broadcast media, digital streaming, social media, podcasts, YouTube, TED Talks—we are virtually bombarded by content from every direction. We know more about food, nutrients, supplements, medicines and side effects than our parents and grandparents did. We read nutritional labels, use microgreens and take micronutrient supplements. We have gadgets and apps galore to tell us what, when and how much to eat, drink or exercise. Our gyms, not just our nutritionists, give us body composition analysis and our personal trainers often plan our diets.

So, is there a need to talk more about food and diet?

My answer is Yes.

And there is a reason for it. Despite this flood of information, content and applications, millions around the world are constantly struggling with minor and major health issues. There are disorders that make people underperform or feel chronically exhausted, or cause regular digestive issues or skin breakouts. On top of this, obesity, gas, bloating, diarrhoea, acid reflux, etc., have become part of our daily existence. Worse, still, many of these issues are simply stepping stones to more serious diseases, such as diabetes, hypertension, heart disease and even cancer.

So clearly, the increased awareness, food category consciousness and growth in healthy eating, despite being positive changes, are not translating into real, lasting health benefits for all. In fact, we are in an age where our young children and youngsters are suffering from adult diseases such as high blood pressure, constipation and diabetes as well as autoimmune diseases such as thyroid disorders, skin and hair issues, and worse still, mental health issues.

According to a Yale public health expert, children in this generation will have a shorter life span than their parents—something that is unprecedented in the history of mankind—as each generation has outlived its previous generation until now.

What is the real reason behind all this? Are we not doing enough? I've seen a broad spectrum of clients saying things like: 'We aren't exercising enough', 'We can't control our cravings', 'We start the day virtuously but give in and eat unhealthy foods towards the end of the workday' or 'We feel like failures'.

Sounds familiar? It probably does to 90 per cent of us.

In response, I would like to say just one thing: **It's NOT Your Fault!**

You feel you can't control your food but actually, it's the other way round . . . your food is controlling you!

We may have more knowledge about food products and be more careful shoppers, but there are modifications to our food universe that are negative. Whether it's altered food ecosystems, levels of pollution, increased use of pesticides or microplastics—and it's very likely a combination of these factors—the fact is that much of what we eat and breathe today leads either to inflammation in the body or addiction, or both.

So, in fact, you are a Victim of these changes, not the Culprit!

Please understand, no one wakes up one morning with diabetes or high blood pressure or cancer or obesity. The development of all such disorders and diseases is progressive. It occurs in stages, many of them almost imperceptible. While not invisible, these staging points are dots that are often not connected until a disease manifests itself. For instance, food cravings (for sugar and starch) are at one end; these could be followed by an imbalance in blood glucose levels and eventually weight gain and belly fat. The end result of which could be full-blown diabetes.

The start and the end points could be anything, but the underlying cause of lifestyle-related diseases actually is chronic **inflammation.**

What Is Inflammation?

Inflammation is an adaptive immune response of the body to foreign bodies, pathogens, toxins or stress.

In short, it is a protective response to battle, sports or other injuries and infections. When you have a fever or a wound is inflamed, you have what is called acute inflammation and it is the result of the body's own healing mechanism being activated. Acute inflammation goes away within hours or days. However, the problem begins when there is **chronic inflammation**. This type of inflammation occurs when the body stays in a state of inflammation for months or often even after the trigger is withdrawn. In fact, chronic inflammation is the starting point of all chronic degenerative diseases, including diabetes, arthritis, heart disease, cancer, Alzheimer's and autoimmune diseases.

What Triggers Chronic Inflammation?

It's a combination of diet, lifestyle and environmental factors. The key culprits that are involved in chronic systemic inflammation are what I call the 4 Gs. These 4 Gs are:

1. Gut
2. Gluten
3. Glucose and
4. Girth

All four of these are intimately connected, to each other and to our bodies, and often the combined effect of these four Gs creates a state of chronic inflammation in the gut—what is referred to as a 'leaky gut', in which toxins from partially digested food move through the gut lining causing other parts of the body to get inflamed. This usually is the root of ill health.

In this book, therefore, I have highlighted the root cause of ill health and disease, which is an imbalanced gut, and the two primary culprits in our modern ecosystem—gluten and grain—along with excessive sugar or glucose.

Part I of this book, **What Is the Problem?** elucidates how central **Gut** function is to health and the factors that influence its effectiveness. I have explained the functioning of the gut and the intimate connection between the condition of the gut and our health and well-being. I have explained how important the gut microbiome is and how the right balance in the microbiome controls virtually all our functionality.

Three chapters are devoted to the other three Gs: they explain what **Gluten** is and why so many people worldwide have 'suddenly' developed an intolerance to this protein so prevalent in our food; the role **Glucose** and other sugars, hidden and visible, play; and how a large **Girth** is both a cause and a consequence of inflammation.

They also elucidate how these inflammatory foods (mentioned in later chapters) are also the most addictive ones, the science behind why consuming them makes you crave more and worsens the addiction—and the inflammation. This is why we continue with incorrect eating habits, in spite of our knowledge of food.

I want to highlight that there is a worrying social non-acceptance among most practitioners of orthodox medicine about acknowledging this connection between the four Gs and ill health. It's not completely surprising, because it is believed that it takes an average of fifteen years for research to get into medical practice. And a lot of the information I am going to give you is from studies that are less than a decade old and some are from currently ongoing research as well.

Part II is about the solution: **What Should We Do?** It is actionable intelligence. Our relationship with food is an intimate one and if we apply the information according to guidelines, it is easy to alter eating habits! What's more, we can do so in a way that can help heal the gut and improve the functioning of its microbiome.

Eating right for oneself is a skill each of us should learn, but it does require understanding. Therefore, this book, dear reader, hopes to empower you with the knowledge that will help you reset your internal health clock. It is simple, once you take the right steps. What follows is an auto mode—changes in the palate, with no struggle, no cravings and less hunger.

You are what you eat, but I take it one step further and say, 'You are what you digest!'

This book is not the latest fad. It is, in fact, a study that I have done with my clients to try and understand the root cause of why our health is the way it is. So you will also get to read impactful stories of people who have made these changes effortlessly and stuck to them. In the process, you will learn to own your health, from the inside out!

Lastly, I have addressed an issue that had taken centre stage in 2020—the pandemic. I talk about how to use dietary intervention and prevention to boost your immune system, so that you can protect your body and fight off incipient infection. The fight against COVID-19 also starts right in the gut.

In fact, the fight for good health starts from the control panel in your belly—quite literally under the belt.

So join in.

PART I

What Is the Problem?

This part highlights the importance of our gut and how it affects every cell of our body. It will help connect all the dots and links the health of our gut to almost all aspects of our health and happiness.

PART I

What Is the Problem?

Chapter I

The Gut Matters

'Always trust your gut; it knows what your head hasn't figured out yet'

—Anonymous

Mr Y, a forty-four-year-old wealth manager with no history of diabetes or hypertension, developed both these and brain fog, and a bad stammer post his COVID-19 vaccination. He also gained 7 kg of weight. With his focus foggy, his work suffered; he was not the sharp man in meetings that he had been until then.

Whether there is stress, joy, depression or anxiety, our bodies feel its impact first in the gut. The need to rush to the washroom when confronted with nerve-wracking events is a simple example. To some extent, we know this, as major events in our lives can be visibly seen to affect the gut. But what we don't know is that these emotions also begin with events in your gut. So central is the gut, not just to the digestive system, but to all the other systems in our bodies, that what happens there potentially impacts every cell and tissue in our body.

When Mr Y consulted me, I found his Vitamin D and B12 levels were low and the lipid profile and liver enzymes were abnormal (which showed how gut flora can shift profoundly post-vaccination). He was put on a regimen that eliminated both gluten and dairy and added gut-healing supplements. In ten days, there was a dramatic improvement; in a month, his symptoms were in complete remission. Sharp as a tack again, he's back at work full-time.

This is not new. About 2500 years ago, the Greek physician Hippocrates, considered the father of modern medicine, declared that all diseases begin in the gut. Hippocrates may not have had the benefit of modern testing, but by observation and analysis, he had concluded that good digestion was a prerequisite for good health. He saw in gut imbalance the beginning of disease and ill health.

Why Is the Gut Crucial?

The gut performs several essential functions in the body and is a critical member of the digestive system, but it does so much more than that. It's also the body's second brain and its healthy activity is also integral to developing a strong immune function. It's also responsible for appetite control and addictions to foods and substances. Plus, it plays a critical role in preventing diabetes, heart diseases and other chronic illnesses. It is the gut that determines the level of absorption of nutrients.

Digestive Function

The human body is a well-honed machine, which functions well even under pressure. During the process of digestion, the constituents in what we eat are broken down, the nutrients are absorbed and the waste is eliminated. Digestion starts in the mouth, leading into the stomach and the gut. It is the beating heart of the digestive system, and the small intestine is a critical part of it. Vital enzymes are secreted in the gut, which help in the breaking down of food into molecules that can be absorbed by the body, and most of the absorption takes place in the gut.

Barrier Function

It is in the small intestine where the food we eat is broken down into molecular form and the nutrients are absorbed into the bloodstream. That is why it is over 20 feet long! So that even those foods that are difficult to digest are metabolized. These particles either get absorbed through the walls of the small intestine into the bloodstream or get carried on through the gastrointestinal tract to be eventually evacuated.

But the gut is also the body's largest interface between the body and the external/outside environment. In an article published online in 2020, Dr Alessio Fasano (Center for Celiac Research and

Treatment and Division of Pediatric Gastroenterology and Nutrition, Massachusetts General Hospital for Children, Boston) connects the dots between the hypothesis Hippocrates made 2500 years ago and a modern scientific understanding of how the gut functions. And the conclusion is inescapable: gut function is critical to good health; when gut function is compromised, the body is set on the path of ill health, disorder and disease.

In the article, Dr Fasano explains that the gut is like a very busy traffic junction, with heavy molecular traffic. And there is constant interaction between the cells of the gut with nutrients, pollutants and the microorganisms in the food molecules and those that reside in the gut. This interactivity is dynamic, far-reaching and is controlled by intercellular tight junctions.

The gut plays a complex double role: it must allow selective permeability of nutrients that the body needs into the internal cells, but it must also prevent the entry of harmful entities. That is the barrier function of the gut and it has a three-ring defence mechanism, which is physical, biological and immunity-based.

The gut function is mediated by our gut flora, also called the microbiome. The gut is host to a large community of good and bad microorganisms. When there is an imbalance in the number of good and bad microorganisms, it leads to inflammation in the gut or leaky gut and opens a doorway to ill health and chronic low-grade systemic inflammation.

Studies show that the gut microbiome is integral to the control of many of the risk factors for cardiovascular disease: nutritional status, inflammation, diabetes, high blood pressure, obesity, cholesterol levels and even the clotting of blood (see box below).

THE PATH TO CHRONIC DISEASE GOES THROUGH THE GUT

- Imbalance in gut flora is clearly linked to obesity and diabetes: it impairs the ability to regulate insulin and store fat
- It leads to inflammation, which is the starting point of all chronic degenerative diseases, from cardiovascular disease to abnormal cholesterol levels and increased clotting tendency
- Gut microbe imbalance is linked to the accumulation of plaque and poor circulation
- Gut flora balance influences the absorption of vitamins and key micronutrients that are critical for insulin metabolism. Low levels of key vitamins can cause hardening of blood vessels
- Food sensitivities and digestive disturbances are directly linked to an unhealthy gut

Many of the disorders and diseases associated with disturbance in the gut have assumed epidemic proportions and have become public health issues (see box 'Disorders on the March', page 9). The data doesn't lie: these figures show an increased prevalence of disorders, mental health issues and more serious diseases. While the underlying causes may be varied and complex, there is compelling evidence that nutrition or simply what we eat is a critical factor in the increased prevalence of mental health and autoimmune disorders as well as the better-known connection with cardiovascular, gastrointestinal and endocrine (hormonal) disorders.

The evidence is growing that the role of the gut microbiome and its optimal functioning impacts virtually every system in the human body. When there is an imbalance in the gut flora, it triggers inflammation and a leaky gut, and then a spiral into ill health. A leaky gut is associated with chronic fatigue, foggy brain, neurological disorders, migraines, food intolerances and allergies, lowered immunity and autoimmunity, skin problems, eczema, psoriasis, hyper-pigmentation, fibromyalgia (muscle pains, joint pains) and migraines. The connection between a leaky gut (increased intestinal permeability) with many diseases is not surprising, but that with obesity is; for a long time, it was believed that obesity *resulted* in inflammation.[1] But now we are in a state where the reverse is also true.

Dr Fasano's study shows that inflammation also results in obesity; it can be the genesis of immunogenic obesity (see more in Chapter VI on girth).

DISORDERS ON THE MARCH

Malnutrition: India bears one of the highest burdens of malnutrition globally; it is the predominant cause of death among children (7.06 lakh deaths in children under the age of five in 2017); 44 per cent of children under the age of five are underweight and malnourished. Women too bear a disproportionate burden of malnutrition: over 50 per cent of women of reproductive age in India are anaemic.[2]

Obesity: The World Health Organization (WHO) has estimated that, by 2025, one in five adults will be obese. The global prevalence of obesity has nearly tripled between 1975 and 2016.

Diabetes: In 2019, India was estimated to have 77 million diabetics. But the prevalence in urban areas was between 11 and 14 per cent, against 3–8 per cent in rural areas.

Cancer: 1300 persons die of cancer in India every day; it's a 6 per cent rise in numbers between 2014 and 2016. Breast cancer incidence has increased from one in twenty-five to one in eight in India. A 2018 report recorded over 1.62 lakh cases in the year and more than 87,000 reported deaths.[3]

Autism: Twenty years ago, one child in 10,000 was autistic; now it's one in fifty-nine.[4]

Autoimmune Disorders: The third most common cause of death in the US. The number of those affected has been doubling every fifteen years since 1945.

Depression and Mental Health: WHO estimated in early 2020 that 264 million people worldwide were afflicted by depression and that one person dies every forty seconds by suicide. The CDC (Centers for Disease Control and Prevention) says that the suicide rate for girls aged fifteen to nineteen doubled from 2007 to 2015. These figures are bound to have increased exponentially with the onset of the coronavirus pandemic and resultant isolationism.

According to a 2012 report in *Lancet*, India has one of the highest suicide rates for youth aged fifteen to twenty-nine. Other reports estimate that one student dies by suicide every hour in India.

Food Allergies: According to the CDC, there has been a 50 per cent increase in food allergies between 1997 and 2011.

What Is the Gut Microbiome?

Our body is not just an enormous collection of cells that make up organs, tissues, nerves, blood vessels, etc. It's also a host—to tens of trillions of microorganisms— bacteria, viruses, fungi and others. Together, these microscopic life forms are called the microbiome and a vast majority of them reside in—you guessed it—the gut! It is estimated that the gut microbiome consists of 10^3–10^4 (trillion) microorganisms; inhabitants that together possess 150 times more genes than the human genome. Put together, these microbes can weigh over 2 kg and should be considered an organ itself. Our health is determined by a complex interplay of their genes, along with the host genome and our environment. Indeed, a fine orchestra!

Gut Microbiome—Our Signature and Our Control Panel

That's why the finely tuned gut microbiome is a unique and complex environment, and no one's microdata is the same as another's. The communities of microbes in the gut are in a state of constant change and they are affected by changes in the host body's condition and environment. A disturbance in the gut microbiome can affect the host's health—it can, therefore, impact every cell, tissue, organ and system—be it cardiac, endocrine, nervous, immune— or even the skin, the largest organ in the body.

These gut microbes are also called gut flora: some of them are beneficial and help the systems of the body function well, but there are others whose activity is harmful. Good bacteria and microbes aid in digestion and absorb nutrients, and this helps us maintain weight and guard against diseases. Other microbes help manufacture essential vitamins that the body cannot make, such as B vitamins, vitamin K and folate.

The Function of the Microbiome

The role played by the gut microbiome in keeping the body healthy or pushing it in the direction of ill health is pivotal. Harmful bacteria disturb the activity of useful bacteria and can create imbalance. This proliferation of bad guys (an imbalance between the good and bad microbes) compromises gut health and begins the development of inflammation and ill health. When there is a disturbance in the balance of gut flora, the microbes produce bacterial toxins called endotoxins like lipopolysaccharides (LPS), which cross over the gut lining, causing a leaky gut and inflammation.

When the gut flora activity begins to work against the host body, it leads to a leaky gut. What causes an imbalance in gut flora? Food that the gut doesn't like. That could be inflammatory grains, proteins, pollutants, pesticides and antibiotics. A single course of antibiotics can significantly disrupt the good and bad gut flora, leaving you with an impaired ability to absorb nutrients and worse, vulnerable against foreign pathogens. The reason: the gut plays a pivotal role in the activity of the immune system. This is why one should be prudent with the intake of any drug or medication.

Immune Function

You might be surprised to learn that more than two-thirds of the immune system is located in the gut. The function of this system is to try and eliminate an invader by creating inflammation and activating antibodies to fight it. The immune system also eliminates the body's own cells when they become diseased.

In order to perform these activities, the cells of the immune system need to be able to tell friends from foes. Gut microbes again play a central role in this:

during digestion, they break down fibre into small molecules that include short-chain fatty acids (SCFAs). These SCFAs influence the immune function of the gut and the activity of the T cells, the informants which help the body recognize which cell is which and decide whether or not to attack.

A disturbance in the gut microbiome directly causes diseases such as inflammatory bowel disease, diarrhoea and many other digestive disorders. It can also be the starting point of several other chronic degenerative diseases outside the gut including asthma, skin diseases, autoimmune diseases and metabolic diseases. Professor Sarkis Mazmanian, professor of microbiology at CalTech, who has studied the effect of gut microbes on health for more than a decade, points out that 'the balance of different bacterial species in the gut can influence whether the immune system becomes activated or not'.

Neurological Function: The Second Brain

But the gut is so much more than the role it plays in digestion, absorption of nutrients and performing the barrier function—though these are essential roles in the body's functioning. The gut is also the body's second brain: about 80 per cent of the human body's neurotransmitters (dopamine, serotonin, tryptophan and others) are secreted in the gut. New research tells us that changes in the gut microbiome can affect the central nervous system, which affects how your brain works. In fact, the most recent studies on Alzheimer's disease are concentrating on healing the gut in order to slow down the progress of this debilitating disease.

So clear is the gut–brain connection that our moods, neurological functionality and mental clarity all depend on the optimal functioning of the gut. Sleep patterns are modulated by the gut. Melatonin, the hormone that controls sleep and wakefulness patterns, was believed to be secreted by the pineal gland; it is, but only 10 per cent; some 90 per cent of melatonin is, in fact, secreted in the gut.

Appetite Control Function

Several appetite-controlling hormones are also secreted in the gut. So, disruption in the gut microbiome determines how much you eat. If you seem to have an insatiable or bottomless-pit type of hunger, or do not feel hungry at all, chances are you need to take a deep dive into the functioning of your gut.

The condition of the gut microbiome also determines our addictions. Addictive foods are inflammatory (see more in the chapters on gluten and glucose), but since they trigger endocannabinoid (a part of the nervous system) receptors in the gut, consuming them makes you want more—and that worsens the addiction. This is a relatively new understanding of our body—that there are these receptors that control our eating behaviour.

For me, as a clinical practitioner, the evidence is compelling. When patients who are following a gluten-free diet have exposure to a grain that either contains gluten or could have been contaminated by some quantity of it, they experience increased hunger, lower energy and disinclination to follow the diet—just like a person trying to de-addict feels when they get on the drug again.

Nutritional Role

Since it is in the gut that absorption of nutrients takes place, the condition of the gut microbiome also helps determine the nutritional status of the host body. Malnutrition, particularly micronutrient malnutrition (common ones include iron, vitamin B12, vitamin D, etc.), is becoming a huge challenge even among the affluent. This is due to the malabsorption of nutrients, as the integrity of the gut lining has been compromised. So, we can say it is likely to be malabsorption, rather than an actual shortage of nutrients.

Despite crores of rupees being spent on anaemia prevention programmes post Independence in India, the number of women and children who remain anaemic remains largely unchanged. So, supplementation is akin to filling a leaky bucket; it only remains full as long as you continue topping up, but if you stop, the level starts dipping again.

Providing Vitamins

Gut microbes also produce vitamin K, important for clotting, and several B- vitamins. It is estimated that up to half of the daily vitamin requirement is provided by the gut bacteria. Recent evidence indicates that vitamin D status may be associated with the gut microbiome and oral supplementation with pro and prebiotics increases circulating vitamin D. It is, therefore, not surprising that in a disturbed gut, deficiencies of these vitamins may easily be explained even among those people who follow a good diet and have plenty of sun exposure.

The Gut's Barrier Function Helps Determine Health Status. How?

The lining of the small intestine is thin, just one layer of cells. This is intentional, to allow for easy absorption. Think of it as a cheesecloth lining a long tube like the intestinal tract, through which very small particles can get through. But if there is inflammation, the lining tears in places, usually at key junction points. This creates a leaky gut or one in which larger molecules of undigested food or foods that are difficult to break down can permeate—and do so before they have been broken down completely into the constituents needed by the body to provide it with its nutritional needs.

These poorly digested particles reach the bloodstream and they can trigger the body to produce antibodies since the body views them as foreign. For example, large molecules of proteins like gluten and dairy are common proteins which cross over the gut lining. Since the body is not familiar with large, partially-digested protein in the blood, antibodies to gluten protein and dairy protein will be produced.

When there is a leaky gut, gluten is usually the primary trigger. Gliadin (part of gluten) triggers zonulin release. Pre-clinical and clinical studies have shown that the zonulin family, a group of proteins modulating gut permeability, is implicated in a variety of inflammatory diseases, including autoimmune, infective, metabolic and tumoral diseases. The resultant tear (permeability) means that several other still-undigested food particles will keep permeating through and result in the formation of antibodies. If the lining tears regularly, the gut becomes leaky and toxins begin to permeate through the thin wall. Studies show that in humans with a leaky gut, intestinal gram-negative bacteria can release an endotoxin called lipopolysaccharide (LPS) into the bloodstream, which is known to increase gut and systemic inflammation.[5]

CHRONIC FATIGUE: A NUTRITIONAL ISSUE

Have low energy levels or feel tired frequently? This is understandable in older people; but when young, physically active people, and even sportspeople report it, it's worrisome.

Chronic fatigue can be ongoing and persistent and gets alleviated with rest. Common symptoms include unrefreshing sleep, muscle and joint pain, frequent sore throat, headache, body ache, forgetfulness, brain fog, irritability and mood swings. Most people resort to stimulants (caffeine, sugar) or pop in supplements (vitamins and proteins) to mask fatigue. Many adapt and live with low energy as a way of life.

But the body is meant to have abundant energy. Faulty diets, a build-up of toxins and inadequate fluid intake slow it down. Other reasons are hormonal imbalances, particularly of the thyroid, deficiencies, intestinal infections (parasites) and food intolerances. Fad dieting, inadequate exercise and chronic stress also contribute.

Optimal levels of energy are only possible when the body gets enough nutrients, unadulterated and chemical-free food, and adequate rest and sleep. Energy is like a bank account: when funds are low, one can apply for an overdraft (read stimulant). But that's a quick fix; you'll feel the physical strain catch up at the end of the day, or the week. Eventually, you have to put something back into the account to pay the energy bill. It's through adequate nutrition that the body can efficiently turn what we eat into energy.

SIBO OR DYSBIOSIS

Imbalance in the gut flora of the small intestines is known as SIBO (small intestinal bacterial overgrowth). It can be a result of food sensitivities, imbalanced diets (high in sugar, preservatives, pesticides and artificial sweeteners), chronic alcohol abuse, excessive medication, hormonal imbalances, stress, sleep deprivation, lack of exercise or simply the ageing process. The symptoms are non-specific; they range from bloating, abdominal distension, abdominal pain or discomfort and diarrhoea to fatigue and weakness.

Long-standing SIBO leads to changes in the intestinal lining, leading to inflammation. It can also lead to candidiasis (an overgrowth of yeast; see more in Chapter V). Other features of SIBO include malabsorption, nutritional deficiencies, metabolic and bone disorders, and neuropathies (numbness and tingling sensation in the extremities). Common deficiencies include iron, and vitamins A, B12, D, E and K. The non-specific nature of SIBO makes it difficult to distinguish and diagnose.

The 5-D Path

An unhappy or leaky gut leads one down the 5-D path of ill health:

- **Dysbiosis,** or gut flora imbalance: When this happens, the gut barrier function gets disrupted and this leads to permeability or a leaky gut. The impaired intestinal barrier means that toxic residue created by poor digestion can leak into the bloodstream. The next step is:
- **Deficiencies,** or malabsorption of nutrients, in which the host body is unable to derive nutrition even from a healthy diet; and
- **Dysfunction,** which can manifest as fatigue, irritability, headaches, low energy, poor sleep, joint and muscle pains, etc. Over time, dysfunction develops into:

- **Disorders,** which can be digestive, psychiatric, neurological, thyroid malfunction, skin or autoimmune; and finally,
- **Diseases,** which could range from heart disease to hypertension, diabetes and cancer.

The human body is a healing machine. But modern lifestyles and exposure to increasing levels of pollution, toxicity and stress keep the gut under constant attack.

Common Signs and Symptoms of a Leaky Gut

- Recurrent digestive complaints
- Milk intolerance
- Liver dysfunction
- Lack of appetite
- Mouth ulcers
- Growth failure
- Difficulty in losing and gaining weight
- Flattened or brittle nails
- Easy bruising
- Anaemia
- Frequent headaches
- Bone and joint paints
- Easy fractures and injuries
- Infertility
- Recurrent miscarriages
- Giddiness, imbalance and vertigo
- Epilepsy
- Numbness and tingling sensation
- Depression
- Anxiety
- Poor attention span
- Itchy blistering rash
- Eczema, psoriasis and vitiligo
- Autoimmunity

Healing the Leaky Gut

But there is good news! A leaky gut is a reversible condition (detailed in Chapter IX, Action Plan). The human body is forgiving and is designed to have an immense capacity to heal itself, and it possesses the resources to do so.

To continue the cloth analogy, ingesting gluten, glucose or excessive sugar, pesticides and other toxins leads to small tears in the lining of the gut. Fortunately, the in-built repair mechanisms begin working, but their efficacy depends on both age and the sheer number of times the rebuilding needs to happen. If the lining tears regularly, the rebuilding slows down. Each repair takes a week to ten days—and even a single cheat-eat or exposure to rogue elements can create another tear. Real and lasting repair needs elimination, but not only of gluten, in case of sensitivity; there needs to be the management of several other factors that contribute to the leaky gut.

Remember the road to good health is paved not only with good intentions but with good intestines.

Chapter II

The 4-G Connectivity

When it comes to the evils assailing our bodies, there are four clear dangers in our modern lifestyles. They are the four Gs: Gut, Gluten, Glucose and Girth. Understand their linkages and you will realize they affect our well-being—or the lack of it!

Gut

As explained in Chapter I, the gut and the gut flora are responsible for our digestion, our appetite regulation ability, how much nutrition we are able to absorb, our physical and emotional well-being—and much more. It's not an exaggeration to say that we are a sum total of our own genes and those of the microbes we host—plus their complex interaction with our environment. If the brain controls our life through the central nervous system, the gut or the second brain determines whether we are well or ill.

So, how can we keep our gut flora in good health? The answer is simple. Our gut microbiome is unique to each of us. If you can customize your gut microbiome to control chronic inflammation, chances are that you are on your way to good health.

You must have noticed that nutritionists these days talk a lot about inflammation. But what actually is inflammation? Please write your definition of inflammation here.

_____

_____

Causes of Inflammation

Inflammation is caused by a combination of varied factors: food sensitivities to gluten, dairy and nuts, imbalanced diets, high sugar intake and the presence of chemical pesticides or preservatives. Even chronic stress, excessive drinking and the frequent use of medicines—especially antibiotics or hormones—can cause inflammation.

Ageing, too, can affect our gut condition. Your gut at age twenty is not the same as at fifty or sixty. Age-related changes in the gut microbiome basically lower the diversity in the range of microbes, in the gut's metabolic ability and in gut motility (the muscular movement in the bowel). Ageing also increases gut permeability. These changes make the older gut frail and more prone to inflammation and illness. If we take care of some of these changes, we can certainly delay ageing, manage illness and prolong longevity. A comprehensive list of thirty-five Ps that we should take into account in taking care of the gut is given in Chapter VII.

Gluten

In the constant battle that the gut and the gut microbiome fight against ill health and disease, what controls the opposing armies of good and bad bacteria is the food we eat.

Grains such as wheat, barley, spelt and rye contain gluten, a mix of two kinds of proteins (glutelins and prolamins). Gluten is what gives flour its elasticity and allows it to be kneaded and made into a variety of products.

But gluten is also the protein responsible for food sensitivities and intolerances (see more in Chapter III, 'Why Wheat-Related Disorders Are on the Rise'). Its presence in the diet can be the spark that sets off inflammatory reactions for those who react adversely to it because of a genetic disposition. Plus, it can lead to a range of disorders, from celiac disease to non-celiac wheat sensitivity (NCWS), wheat allergy and the itchy and blistery skin condition dermatitis herpetiformis— celiac disease outside the gut.

According to studies, nearly 30 per cent of people believed they were gluten-sensitive. There is also a sizeable number of silent, asymptomatic patients whose sensitivity is only discovered by chance, or the sensitivity appears outside the gut and you can see other manifestations like skin disorders. With gluten sensitivity, you may experience difficulty in losing weight, bloating, digestive disorders, obesity or the other end of the spectrum—you may be morbidly thin and unable to gain weight.

Not only does gluten cause adverse effects but it is also morphine-like in its addictiveness. The reason is that when gluten is digested, it's broken down into gluten exorphins, which are opiate-like proteins that imitate the effect that opiates have on the body. These highly addictive components perpetuate our craving for excess food. They also explain the need for more and more.

The good news is that it is possible to break the vicious cycle of gluten inflammation and addiction. When I advise my clients to begin using alternative flours like millets or pulse flours, they feel better, lighter, more energetic, and their biomarkers (blood sugar levels, cholesterol levels, etc.) improve dramatically (see case studies in Chapter XIII).

Glucose and Sugars

For decades, health practitioners have talked about fats and cholesterol as the villains of ill health and heart disease. The fats were a strict no-no as diet plans grew around their exclusion and an entire medical and wellness industry went around believing that cholesterol reduction was *the* goal.

All this while, sugars stayed quietly in the background, hiding their presence in food like breakfast cereals, bakery biscuits or in the form of desserts, candy chocolate and even some health-food bars. Sugars even found their way into sauces, juices, tonic water and dressings. Research suggests that billions of dollars have been spent by the sugar lobby globally for governments and doctors to NOT talk of sugar as a major contributor to ill health and to keep the fats and cholesterol association the only thing we talk about.[1]

But though a diet that is high in animal protein and unhealthy fats is not a healthy one, sugar worsens the lipid (fats) profile, increasing the levels of low-density lipoprotein (LDL, the bad cholesterol) and triglycerides. It also lowers levels of the good cholesterol—high-density lipoprotein (HDL). A poor lipid profile can indeed increase the risk of heart disease, but the role of sugar remains unpublicized. Excessive sugar may also be associated with insulin resistance and eventually lead to diabetes.

Sugar was only associated with diabetes. Its connection with dysbiosis (by fueling unfriendly colonies of yeast and candida) is only recently being recognized. As is the villainous role played by hidden and invisible sugar in our diet (see more in Chapter V, 'Glucose: The Dark Side'). It is this aspect of sugar that provokes inflammation, starting from dysbiosis and leaky gut, and resulting in chronic inflammation.

Girth

Our bodies should have *some* fat. But how much of it, and where it is stored, is crucial. It's all about location (more about this in Chapter VI).

Visceral fat is the kind that's stored deep in the abdomen (stomach region)—and that is the one you don't want. It's wrapped around the abdomen and its internal organs such as the kidneys, pancreas and liver. If visceral fat is more than optimal, it can adversely impact cardiometabolic health by increasing inflammation. The higher the amount of visceral fat, the greater the risk for many inflammatory diseases like diabetes, high blood pressure, heart disease and even skin disorders.

The existence of visceral fat is not always obvious, though having a big belly is a good indicator of its presence. Usually, the bigger the girth (belly measurement), the higher the level of visceral fat. However, we also see otherwise slim people with large bellies, which is indicative of the presence of visceral fat. These are the 'thin fat people'. Such obesity is referred to as abdominal obesity, truncal obesity or apple-shaped obesity. General obesity is called pear-shaped obesity.

Combined Effect of the Four Gs

The combined effect of the four Gs has the most profound impact on inflammation in the body, leading to a leaky gut. This further results in malnutrition or malabsorption of nutrients, propelling the body towards ill health.

In order to begin the journey towards better health, one needs to understand how each one of the Gs works and how to break the cycle of connectivity that can cause disorder and chaos.

Only then can you begin to heal the gut. And remember, a healthy gut means a healthy body!

Chapter III

Why Wheat-Related Disorders Are on the Rise

Is gluten the new fat? Or is 'gluten-free' the new fad?

I have been asked this question many times. Why has a grain that has been eaten for thousands of years suddenly become problematic? One of the main reasons that most people, including most medical professionals, find it difficult to understand wheat sensitivity is the simple, logical fact that our ancestors lived—and indeed thrived—on wheat, barley and other ancient grains. Since Biblical times, grain cultivation has been integral to civilizations.

So why has wheat become the bogeyman of our diet? Wheat is not the only culprit (there are other grains that contain gluten), although it's the biggest offender because of its wide presence across food products. We don't really *eat* much rye, spelt or barley (barley is the main constituent of beer, though).

What people the world over eat is either bread, pasta or rotis and naans (all made from wheat flour of varying degrees of refining).

Wheat and Health

Wheat's connection with ill health is historic and has had many manifestations (see Fig. 1). It's one of the top eight allergens along with dairy, eggs, soya, nuts, tree nuts, shellfish and fish; its ingestion can lead to wheat allergy (fairly uncommon) in some cases, celiac disease or a typical itchy skin rash called dermatitis herpetiformis; and now, there's a whole new entity under the umbrella of non-celiac wheat-related disorders (NCWS or non-celiac wheat sensitivity). But until about sixty-odd years ago, many of these disorders affected a small percentage of the population (celiac disease is estimated to affect about 1 per cent of people in India).[1] That's partly the reason why the medical fraternity and the public are divided between those who believe eating wheat is damaging to our gut health and those who think that we can't blame something that has been integral to our diets for ages.

But what we see happening since the 1960s is that the incidence of gut reactions to wheat is far more widespread (celiac disease has increased more than fourfold in this period), across cultures and geographies.[2]

Actually, there need not be a divide at all!

Research reveals that the dramatic increase in celiac disease and other wheat-related disorders took place when **new wheat varieties** were introduced into our

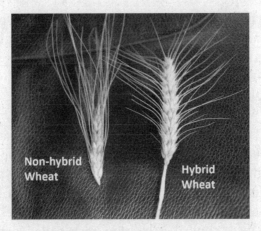

Fig. 1

diet. The 'wheat' we eat today is so different from its ancestor plants that it's not surprising our gut reaction to it is so different from that of our forefathers'! We are also eating new varieties of other crops, from corn to soya. Hybrid varieties are ubiquitous in the food chain—and their effects on our digestive and other systems are not yet fully understood.

Take wheat, because it is used in food products across cultures. The game changer has been changes in the plant variety itself. Sophisticated hybridization techniques (called transgene hybrid systems) were used to produce new strains of modern, transgenic wheat. While these were supposed to be high in yield and disease-resistant, some strains have also had the undesirable effect of promoting ill health.[3] It is possible that tampering with a known allergen potentiated its immunogenicity.

These variants were introduced by importing wheat supplies in the 1960s. The number of varieties has also grown exponentially since then, from a few kinds of wild grass to over 20,000 varieties! What we get on our tables also bears little resemblance to the traditional varieties in their genetic make-up. We can easily see that since these new varieties came in, there has been an exponential increase in the incidence of heart disease, diabetes and obesity, cancer and other autoimmune diseases, and the numbers have continued to grow, despite increased use of medical and lifestyle interventions.

I'll try and explain. Wheat was first cultivated about 10,000 years ago, in the 'Neolithic Revolution', as humans transitioned from hunter–gatherers to agriculturists. The first wild wheat, called 'einkorn', the great ancestor plant, has the simplest genetic code of all wheat, containing only fourteen chromosomes. Not long after the einkorn variety began to be cultivated, another variety, 'emmer', developed. Emmer was a combination of einkorn and an unrelated wild grass, and the genetic make-up became a little more complex, with twenty-eight chromosomes. So, the earliest forms of wheat, einkorn and emmer were diploid (having two sets of seven chromosomes) and tetraploid (having four sets of seven chromosomes).

For many centuries, these varieties, which yielded a flour denser than what we use, reigned supreme. In fact, the Egyptians are credited with the discovery of making the dough rise by using yeast.

While not exactly native to India, wheat travelled to the subcontinent via the Silk Road from central Asia, over 8000 years ago. Today, it's the second-largest crop in the country, after rice. And while we do grow the 14-chromosome emmer and durum varieties, over

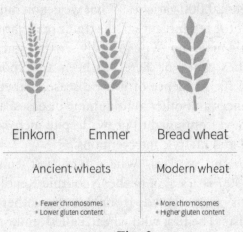

Einkorn   Emmer   Bread wheat

Ancient wheats   Modern wheat

• Fewer chromosomes   • More chromosomes
• Lower gluten content   • Higher gluten content

Fig. 2

85 per cent of the cultivated wheat in the subcontinent is of the 42-chromosome hexaploid variety.

Our native crops were rice, millets and barley. Lentils such as black gram and moong were integral to Indian agriculture for thousands of years. Pulses (chickpeas, kidney beans and black-eyed beans) were domestic crops in the Indus Valley civilization.

New-Generation Grain

A few thousand years ago, modern wheat, which is hexaploid, made its first appearance via another mating process. It had a higher yield, so it soon took over. Currently, about 95 per cent of the wheat grown worldwide is hexaploid (which contains six sets of chromosomes, a total of forty-two). Most bread wheat is hexaploid, and most of the remaining 5 per cent is tetraploid durum pasta wheat.

But the wheat we eat today bears little resemblance to even the original hexaploid plant that developed organically. American agronomist Norman Borlaug (who spearheaded the Green Revolution and received the Nobel Peace Prize for his efforts to save people from starvation by exponentially increasing the food supply), developed semi-dwarf, high-yield, disease-resistant wheat varieties through his agricultural research in Mexico. He also led the introduction of these varieties into Mexico, Pakistan and India, nearly doubling the yields in India and Pakistan. India witnessed a major increase in agricultural productivity in 1965 with the advent of the Green Revolution. This turned the country's agricultural regions into bread baskets with a major increase in the productivity of food and cash crops like wheat, rice, pulses, jute, sugarcane, tea, cotton and so on. The productivity of wheat and rice crops registered a threefold increase during this period.

The changes rung in by the Green Revolution certainly fed people and alleviated hunger—but at the cost of malnutrition and even the advent of new diseases. Borlaug's work has also faced opposition from environmentalists and nutritionists who consider genetic cross-breeding to have negative health effects. Especially in a protein known to have inherent immunogenic effects, unlike rice and other crops. To make wheat disease-resistant, maximize yield and make it even easier to thresh, the hybrid varieties were created—with hardly any or completely inadequate food safety studies on the immune response in humans.[4]

Further tinkering with the plant has concentrated on modifying the plant genome to create flours that are better for baking, so they are used to make an ever-increasing variety of products. And we are consuming more and more of these products: from basic ones such as bread, naan and roti to processed forms such as burgers, croissants, pizzas, pastries and cakes.

Is modern wheat higher in gluten? It may not be. But while the **total gluten content** of the grain may not have increased, the **expression of the immunogenic fractions** has increased, and research suggests this is due to the hybridization process. This generation of wheat is so different from earlier forms of the wheatgrass, it may as well have been from Mars! The newer varieties are highly immunogenic (the ability of a substance to provoke an immune response) compared to earlier varieties.[5]

Einkorn Compared to Modern Wheat

Einkorn	Modern Wheat
Never hybridized	Hybridized naturally and commercially multiple times
Never had chemical or genetic technologies used to produce	Genetic and chemical technologies used to raise production
A genome for gluten—a different type of gluten that does not even register on the ELISA test for gluten	D genome of gluten, which is the main contributor of gluten sensitivities

Diploid—only two simple sets of chromosomes	Tetraploid—six sets of chromosomes
High in vitamins and low in dangerous heavy metals	

S. No.	Properties	Ancient	Modern
1.	Chromosomes	Diploid (14 chromo-somes)	Hexaploid (42 chromo-somes)
2.	Wheatgrass	Tall	Dwarf
3.	Yield	Low yield	High yield
4.	Pest	Prone	Resistant
5.	Pesticide	Sensitive	Resistant
6.	Gluten	Low	High
7.	Nutrient values Magnesium Calcium Iron Copper	High High High High High	Low Low Low Low Low
8.	Variety	Soft	Hard

The two main components of wheat gluten are glutenin and gliadin, with the latter being more abundant. Dr William Davis, author of *The Wheat Belly*, postulates in an article called 'The Gliadin Effect' that gliadin in present-day wheat is different in its composition of amino acids than the gliadin before 1960. And this is due to the genetic process used to create the higher yield varieties. He points out that gliadin breaks down into polypeptides called exorphins in the intestinal tract. These exorphins cross the blood–brain barrier and bind to the opiate receptors in the body—and increase appetite, induce behavioural changes such as outbursts and inattentiveness in children, autism and so on. Gliadin provokes a stronger immunogenic response and increases intestinal permeability (leaky gut).

Wheat also contains a lectin called wheat germ agglutinin (WGA), which has been shown to interfere with protein digestion and increase gut permeability. Lectins are a type of protein that chooses and binds to carbohydrates on cell membranes. They can trigger an inflammatory response, causing gastrointestinal symptoms like cramping, bloating, flatulence, hyperacidity, diarrhoea, nausea and vomiting. They are also implicated in food intolerances, and inflammatory and autoimmune conditions such as rheumatoid arthritis. Many food allergies are actually immune system reactions to lectins.

Lectins in food protect the seeds from pests and insects. The genetic modification of plants created a fluctuation in lectin content to develop pest-resistant varieties. Our bodies do not digest lectins but create antibodies against them! Scientific literature shows that dietary lectins disrupt intestinal flora by reducing natural killer cells, the important defences against viruses and other invaders, thereby affecting our immune functions. They are also pro-inflammatory and contribute to leaky gut.[6]

WHY DID ONLY WHEAT BECOME IMMUNOGENIC?

- While we do not know the exact reasons, one possibility is that wheat is a known allergen. Historically, wheat allergy and celiac disease have been recognized as health issues for over a century.
- When a known allergen is further manipulated by making chromosomal changes in the genetic material (done during the Green Revolution) without long-term safety trials, the emergence of a super immunogenic seed is not hard to imagine.
- Besides higher yields, it was designed to withstand higher pesticide load; this allowed heavy use of glyphosate and other weedicides, leading to dysbiosis, leaky gut and chronic inflammation.

Research papers have said that 'the Green Revolution led to drastic changes in the structure of wheat gluten proteins during hybridization' and that the 'outbreaks of the new gluten and wheat sensitivity syndromes have taken place during the very same period of time in which thousands of new wheat hybrids were introduced into human foods'. They also cite a study that revealed, '14 new gluten proteins . . . in the offspring that were not present in either parent wheat'.[7]

In another study, the effects of kamut, a recently rediscovered ancient variant of wheat (which has about double the total gluten and a-gliadin content of modern wheat) were compared with those of modern wheat varieties. The kamut replacement diet showed a reduction in six biomarkers for inflammation and in both total and LDL cholesterol.

Our Gut Microbiome Has Also Changed[8]

The period since modern wheat varieties were introduced has also coincided with a huge increase in processed foods. Researchers believe increased consumption of processed foods has compromised the body's ability to digest the proteins in wheat and dairy. It is a fact that both gluten and a-gliadins are hard to digest, but there are microbes throughout the gastrointestinal tract that help break them down. So, the balance of the microbes in the gut assumes centre stage—if there is an imbalance, it can lead to wheat and dairy sensitivity.

Other experts also point to the fact that most grains are grown with increased use of fertilizers and pesticides (see paragraphs on the glyphosate connection). The hybrid variety of wheat was, in fact, designed to withstand the heavy use of pesticides. Is it surprising then that the incidences of gluten sensitivity have increased?

Dairy: Neither a Villain nor a Hero

Now let's look at dairy. It is estimated that 50 per cent of those who are gluten-sensitive are also dairy intolerant. My own clinical practice does not contradict these estimates, but there are no simple answers on dairy products. There are several components of dairy that could be neutral, beneficial or downright harmful—and their effect varies from person to person. Keeping a log of one's own symptoms is really the best way to find out.

That milk is a good source of nutrients is true. Mother's milk, in particular, is a high-energy delivery system—and helps babies grow exponentially. In adults, however, drinking milk is not always productive. Milk protein consists of about 80 per cent casein (this content is intensified in cheese). But casein shares some similarities with some components of gluten, and it, too, can cause a histamine or allergic response, such as increased asthma, headaches and gastrointestinal issues. That's why people sensitive to gluten have an increased risk of being intolerant to casein—in fact, research shows that half of those who have celiac disease are also sensitive to dairy.

Whey is a blend of other proteins and hormones present in milk, and includes immunoglobins and insulin-like growth factors. This means that dairy products cause the body to release large amounts of insulin. In those with metabolic syndrome (see chapter on glucose), this can lead to insulin resistance, which can trigger inflammation. Whey protein powder may alter the microbiome negatively. Either way, if an individual wants to improve insulin sensitivity, it's best to limit the amount of dairy taken.

THE CALCIUM CONUNDRUM

'But what about Calcium?' This question comes from the perception that milk is high in calcium and so is needed to build strong, healthy bones.

Fallacy 1: Bone-building depends solely on calcium
Fallacy 2: Your calcium *intake* is the only thing that matters, and
Fallacy 3: Dairy is the only good source of calcium.

Fact: Bone development depends on many factors: nutrition, sun exposure, exercise and hormone levels. Yes, calcium is important, but so are three critical vitamins: vitamin C, K and D. As are minerals such as magnesium and phosphorus. To build strong bones, one needs:

- to avoid inflammatory grains and legumes that contain compounds which limit the absorption of essential minerals;
- nutrient-dense foods, especially dark, leafy greens;

- to ensure optimum vitamin D, and adequate dairy fat to ensure its absorption; and
- regular weight-bearing exercises to improve bone density.

Consumption of dairy also increases the levels of IGF-1 (insulin-like growth factor 1), another growth enhancer. IGF-1 helps children grow but has been associated with the development of certain cancers (such as those of the breast, prostate and colon).[9]

And then there is lactose, or milk sugar.

Many people lose the ability to digest lactose with age and report bloating, gastrointestinal upsets and similar issues. Lactose intolerance is quite common. And in such individuals, even the consumption of small amounts can cause an imbalance in the gut flora. Such people could be sensitive to casein and other dairy protein as well.

Take the case of Shruti Arora. A young mother of thirty-three, with a three-month-old baby, she was frustrated with her health and her weight. Her haemoglobin, magnesium, ferritin, vitamin B and D3 levels were low. Plus, she couldn't sleep a wink because the baby was colicky and cranky day and night. She was the patient, but it was obvious her problems were also connected with the discomfort her baby was in. I soon realized that both mother and child had to be treated, if the poor mother's problems had to be resolved.

Her symptoms included polycystic ovary syndrome (PCOS), acne, dark pigmentation and a hypothyroid condition. She had had a C-section and had gained 23 kg. She told me she was constantly hungry, had hyperacidity, sweet and salt cravings and was gassy.

I could see that antibodies to some foods had crossed over the placental barrier and affected the baby in the womb. My goal was to treat both the mother and the child. Because of her autoimmune condition (hypothyroidism), I asked her to remove inflammation-inducing grains and suggested a simple switch to jowar (sorghum) roti.

The effect on the baby was immediate: within a day, the colic had disappeared. But that was when she mentioned her baby was also severely constipated (he would pass stool once in four or five days, and sometimes once in ten to twelve days!). I asked her—to her utter shock—to stop dairy products. She replied that her mother-in-law wouldn't allow a lactating mother to swear off milk. I suggested she explain that milch animals don't drink milk, they eat greens. That worked, and by the second day, the baby was pooping ten to twelve times a day and soon came down to two or three times a day. The baby's distress also stopped and the mother could rest, transforming both lives.

This was not just a case of proving that antibodies to inflammatory foods cross over the placenta but also cross through breast milk. And she was her own case control because as soon as she gave in to the temptation of a few bites of naan or cake, she could see the immediate effects of it on the infant.

Slowly her other issues like pigmentation, hypothyroidism and accompanying problems also vanished!

Is Butter Better?

Where milk scores, however, is in its fat content: organic, pasteurized milk butter particularly when it is in the form of ghee or clarified butter and cream.

Studies show that full-fat dairy promotes better health. Butter has hardly any of the protein fractions present in full-fat milk but does contain other compounds that promote health (vitamin K2, vitamin A, etc.)

And when butter is clarified into ghee, it removes milk proteins. Fermentation helps too: when milk is fermented, the bacterial action involved in the process has broken down most of the proteins and lactose—improving dairy tolerance. And the bacteria themselves help maintain the gut flora balance. But the tolerance varies from person to person, so it has to be analysed by observing reactions and symptoms.

Giving Up Dairy?

The rise in food intolerances means that the number of those who are eliminating wheat or dairy (or both) from their diets is growing. This is also due to the fact that veganism is a fast-growing segment (some reports in the UK suggest a whopping 360 per cent growth in veganism).[10]

But are the alternatives truly healthy?

Some alternatives that are ruling the supermarket shelves are soy, almond and other nut milks and even grain milks like rice, oats, etc. There are non-dairy creamers available as well—or so they claim. Whether they are actually non-dairy is questionable—and these substitute milks may not necessarily be healthier either.

Soy milk contains sodium caseinate and hydrogenated soyabean oil. Casein is a milk protein, so it is not really dairy-free! And hydrogenated oils (also present in non-dairy creamers) contain toxic trans fats, which are known to promote inflammation in the body. Creamers also contain dehydrated high-fructose corn syrup (HCFS: see more in Chapter V, on FODMAPs), a form of sugar that has been linked to insulin resistance, obesity and diabetes. Many of these alternative products also contain non-food, chemical additives.

The logic to apply when choosing alternatives is simple:

- It's not enough to eliminate substances that you don't tolerate well—the substitutes need to be healthy ones.
- If the substitutes are loaded with processed or toxic ingredients, it will cause increased inflammation.
- A gluten-free diet (GFD) is counter-productive if the gluten-free alternatives are processed and/or high in other starches.
- Removing animal proteins and replacing them with processed, starchy or sugary vegetarian alternatives is not a recipe for good health.
- A healthy diet consists of fresh vegetables that are rich in plant protein, seasonal fruits, and healthy

whole grains and pulses. For dairy alternatives, see the next section.

- Last but not least, read the ingredient labels: the thumb rule is, 'If they are difficult to pronounce, don't consume them'; they obviously contain chemicals you are better off without.

Alternatives to Cow Milk

The goat is known as the poor man's cow. But in fact, the nutritive value of goat milk is not significantly different from cow milk[11] and the smaller fat globules mean it's more easily digestible.

Once thought to be useful sustenance for denizens of the desert, camel milk is now known to be as much as three times richer in iron and vitamin C content compared to cow or buffalo milk. It is also high in proteins with antimicrobial potential and is a good source of minerals such as zinc, magnesium, potassium and others—all of which help immune function. It is high in B vitamins, contains essential fatty acids that aren't present in cow or buffalo milk and is low in cholesterol. It can, therefore, also play a protective role in coronary artery disease. The application of natural camel milk products to treat autism-spectrum disorders is growing around its benefits in autistic children.[12]

It's low in lactose and is a useful substitute for those who are lactose-intolerant. It's a natural source of alpha-hydroxy acid, which helps keep skin young and supple. There is also anecdotal evidence that it's high in insulin and insulin-like substances that can help manage diabetes. A 2005 study in Bikaner,[13] in fact, found that its consumption helped patients with type 1 diabetes (in which people cannot produce insulin). This property of camel milk has been linked to the fact that camels graze on natural desert vegetation, including salty herbs and neem leaves. Camel milk is saltier, need not be cooked and has a higher shelf life, making it useful for processing into cheese, butter, buttermilk and other fermented dairy products.

The Glyphosate Connection

Glyphosate is the active ingredient in the herbicide Roundup, which is applied to the leaves of plants to kill pests and its sodium salt form is used to regulate plant growth and ripen fruit. Since it was introduced in 1974, glyphosate-based herbicides' application has increased approximately a hundredfold. Significant amounts of wheat crops are treated with this toxic chemical. It is estimated to be the most widely produced herbicide in the world. Though many experts believe it to be safe, the rise in the use of Roundup has dovetailed with an exponential rise in the incidence of cancer, autism, cardiac disease and digestive tract disorders.

Several other diseases associated with glyphosates include diabetes, obesity, asthma, Alzheimer's, amyotrophic lateral sclerosis (ALS), cancer and Parkinson's disease. Its association with autism is also emerging (see more in the chapter on the thirty-five Ps). There are studies that show that these disorders and diseases can be traced through pathways damaged by glyphosate.[14]

EFFECT OF THE GREEN REVOLUTION ON CANCER

- The Green Revolution was based on the introduction of high-yield varieties—but also the application of chemical fertilizers and pesticides. Consumption of fertilizers grew from 78,000 tons in 1965–66 to 2.5 million tons in 2009–10 and pesticides from 154 metric tons in 1954 to 88,000 metric tons in 2000–01.

- Punjab, the hub of the Green Revolution, saw the biggest increase in the production of foodgrains as well as cash crops, such as cotton. But the incidence of cancer too went up. A 2013 report by the Department of Health and Family Welfare indicates that cancer prevalence in the Malwa region of Punjab is 1089/million, higher than the national average (800/million) and that in other Punjab regions (Majha is 674/million and Doaba is 881/million).

- Malwa is called India's Cancer Capital, with 46 per cent of the total cancer deaths in Punjab. The study pointed to factors related to pesticide exposure as causes, rather than alcohol intake and tobacco smoking as the probable cause of the DNA change and damage.

- The explanation: the farmers were overusing pesticides and not handling the toxic chemicals safely.

Key Takeaways

The arguments can go back and forth, but the salient points remain:

- The incidence of wheat sensitivities has increased exponentially over the last few decades.
- Even if an exact causal relationship cannot be established, this increase has coincided with the mass development of transgenic varieties of wheat.
- Ancient forms of wheat as well as fermented and sprouted forms seem to be easier to digest and do not spark off severe gastrointestinal tract symptoms.
- Current diets, which include all kinds of processed foods as well as a wider variety of wheat products, have an adverse effect on the diversity of the gut microbiome—and, by extension, the ability to break down foods that are hard to digest, such as gluten.

Chapter IV

Wheat and Weight

Like many other cereals, wheat is a high carbohydrate content, high glycaemic index (GI) staple that has the potential to create sharp spikes in blood sugar levels. When it is added to other high GI foods such as desserts and fried snacks that frequently appear on our tables, the propensity to increased girth or obesity—or both—increases, along with diabetes, abnormal cholesterol levels and coronary artery disease.

This effect has worsened because of the growth in the consumption of products that contain highly refined wheat flour namely, maida. The processing of wheat even for atta robs it of fibre and important nutrients. The poor nutritional levels of the flour we eat is a major contributor to the increase in girth today.

It's addictive!

As I said in Chapter II, we cannot forget the addictive nature of the gluten protein, which promotes loss of the appetite control mechanism. Wheat ranks right there with opiates in its effect on the brain. As I explained, when gluten is broken down in the body, some of the resultant polypeptides can cross into the brain and combine with the morphine receptor. That means creating a high and then the experience of withdrawal. It also increases the appetite—for more. The pleasure centres keep demanding it. In addition, there are eight appetite-controlling hormones secreted in the gut. The negative impact of gluten and wheat causes a state of imbalance and disrupts the synthesis of these hormones. Appetite dysregulation is an obvious outcome of this.

Thankfully, going completely off it can and does promote physical well-being and a big improvement in mood—quite apart from the bonus of reducing the wheat belly. With the increasing recognition of toxicity and ill health associated with modern wheat, farmers, agriculturists, the food industry and health professionals need to understand gluten-related sensitivity. The exponential growth of the gluten-free market in the last few years globally cannot be ignored as a food fad alone.

If Not Wheat, Barley or Rye, Then What?

Just rice? Of course not! Thankfully, the grain landscape is not that bleak. In fact, India offers perhaps the widest variety of alternative cereals—from a range of millets (ragi, bajra, jowar), to traditional fasting grains such as kuttu (buckwheat), samak (barnyard millet) and singhara (water chestnut), to lentils and their flours. These are gluten-free, nutritionally dense and better tolerated by the gut. Being devoid of gluten, they facilitate better absorption. Nutrient levels in general are comparable and even better in some. Example: ragi is rich in calcium and iron, compared to wheat.

Celiac Disease: Prime Gluten-Related Disorder

Celiac disease is an autoimmune disease of the gut, involving IgA and IgG antibodies that form against gliadin but does not involve mast cells or IgE (i.e., non-IgE mediated allergy). Sometimes, sensitivity to wheat can be confused with celiac disease (we will address this sensitivity a little later in this chapter), especially since both disorders involve a reaction to gluten.

Types of Celiac Disease

- Typical Celiac Disease
- Atypical Celiac Disease
- Silent Celiac Disease
- Potential Celiac Disease
- Latent Celiac Disease
- Transient Gluten Intolerance
- Dermatitis Herpetiformis

However, celiac disease is not the same thing as an IgE-mediated wheat allergy. It is a condition in which the individual is intolerant to gluten for life. Eating food that contains gluten causes an immune reaction in the small intestine that can damage the villi on the gut lining (which are rather like shags on a carpet) and lower its ability to absorb essential nutrients. But both the diagnosis of celiac disease and its dietary management are challenging, for a variety of reasons: awareness is limited, symptoms can be diverse, non-specific or absent, food options are restrictive and food labelling inadequate.

Untreated, celiac disease can be fatal. But with an incidence estimated to be about 1 in 100 in India, consistent with the global average, over 95 per cent of sufferers remain undiagnosed. The disease occurs globally (Japan is an exception), has no socio-economic boundaries and can occur at any age, although the average age of diagnosis is over forty-five years.

Symptoms of Celiac Disease

Diarrhoea	Bone problems
Gastrointestinal disturbances	Skin problems
	Infertility
Growth problems	Mouth ulcers
Anaemia	Numbness
Weight loss	Behavioural problems
Lethargy	Mental health issues
Tiredness	

Typical symptoms: Diarrhoea, gastrointestinal disturbances like bloated stomach, flatulence, pain, constipation, nausea and vomiting. It can also cause growth problems, like stunting in children, and anaemia.

Atypical Symptoms: The rest have atypical symptoms such as weight loss, lethargy, tiredness, skin problems, osteoporosis or muscle cramps, infertility, mouth ulcers and numbness or behavioural issues such as depression, anxiety, irritability or poor school performance in schoolchildren. For every celiac with digestive disorders, there are eight who have none and symptoms outside the gut.

One atypical presentation of celiac disease is dermatitis herpetiformis, a chronic inflammatory skin condition that manifests in the form of an itchy, red, blistering rash that usually appears on the outer surfaces of the elbows, knees and buttocks, or on the face and scalp. Such symptoms make diagnosis difficult and can lead to more threatening maladies. People with this type of hidden celiac disease are at a higher risk of developing severe malnutrition, non-specific ill health and if the disease remains undiagnosed, even malignancies. Celiac disease, in any case, increases the risk of other autoimmune disorders (like Type 1 diabetes, rheumatoid arthritis, Hashimoto's thyroiditis, psoriasis, multiple sclerosis, systemic lupus erythematosus (SLE), vitiligo and lichen planus, to name a few.

It is clearly a multi-symptom, multi-system disease, which needs to be looked at far more closely than it is at present.

What Causes Celiac Disease?

The answers are not clear. We know that it is an autoimmune hereditary condition and involves a complex interaction of genetic and environmental factors. Early infant feeding practices (lower levels of breastfeeding and early introduction of gluten) may be contributing factors. Breast milk provides the immature immune system with antibodies and protects the gastrointestinal system, strengthens the intestinal lining and improves its barrier function. So, there is a genetic factor and an environmental trigger (in this case, wheat); together, they allow celiac disease to manifest. The fact that there is hardly any evidence of celiac disease in predominantly rice-eating nations like Japan points towards gluten as the environmental trigger.

Unlike in a wheat allergy, those with celiac disease also need to avoid rye, barley, and gluten-containing oats in addition to wheat (see Chapter X, box: 'A Grain of Sense', for cross-reactivity). People who suspect they may have celiac disease should consult a gastroenterologist.

Associated Conditions

General	• Developmental delay in children (cognitive impairment • Chronic fatigue syndrome • Obesity (rarely seen) • IgA deficiency • Fibromyalgia (chronic, widespread pain) • Candida albicans (fungal infection) • Thrombocytopenic purpura (life-threatening, multisystem disorder)
Gastrointestinal	• Dyspepsia (difficulty in digestion) • Gastrointestinal bleeding • Irritable bowel syndrome, improved with gluten exclusion • Intestinal permeability • Colitis (microscopic/lymphocytic) • Cancer, lymphoma

Manifestations of malabsorption	• Nutritional deficiencies, particularly iron, folic acid, vitamins B12 and D • Casein or cow's milk intolerance
Other autoimmune disorders	• Addison's disease • Autism • Crohn's disease • Down's or Turner's syndrome • Sjogren's syndrome (autoimmune disease characterized by abnormal production of extra antibodies in the blood that are directed against various tissues of the body) • Multiple sclerosis • Scleroderma (autoimmune disease characterized by hardening in skin or organs)
Psychiatric	• Attention deficit hyperactivity disorder (ADHD) • Schizophrenia (chronic, severe brain disorder)

Neurological	• Unexplained neurological complaints (especially neuropathies, memory impairment, epilepsy or muscular stiffness) • Brain damage • Migraine • Lupus
Haematological	• Anaemia
Reproduction	• Infertility • Impotency • Recurrent miscarriages
Renal	• Kidney disease
Endocrine	• Growth hormone deficiency • Pancreatic disorders • Diabetes (insulin-dependent with poor control) • Thyroid disease (hypo/hyperthyroidism)
Hepatic system	• Liver disease • Liver enzyme disturbances, especially autoimmune hepatitis, non-alcoholic steatohepatitis (NASH), primary biliary cirrhosis (PBC), primary sclerosing cholangitis (PSC)

Cardiovascular	• Heart failure
Musculoskeletal	• Arthritis—juvenile and adult • Ataxia (difficulty in coordination)
Skin	• Psoriasis (red, scaly patches on the skin) • Dermatitis herpetiformis
Others	• Sarcoidosis (inflammatory disease that may affect any organ or system in the body) • Tuberculosis • Systemic inflammatory reactions (multiple organ dysfunction)

Major Complications Arising from Celiac Disease

- Anaemia
- Skeletal problems:
  - Short stature
  - Dental enamel hypoplasia (incomplete formation of dental enamel)
  - Osteopenia/Osteoporosis (low bone mineral density)
- Neurological problems:
  - Gluten ataxia (loss of coordination due to gluten sensitivity)

- Infertility
- Liver disease
- Intestinal lymphomas

Individuals at Risk of Developing Complications

- People with no gastrointestinal symptoms (silent/ atypical), as they do not show symptoms on consuming gluten
- People suffering from dermatitis herpetiformis
- Adolescents and teenagers who exhibit rebellious behaviour, especially on restrictions
- Those who eat out frequently are exposed to contamination

Has Celiac Disease Increased or Are We Diagnosing More?

There are some who suggest that the exponential growth in numbers is due to improved diagnosis. But a study conducted by the Mayo Clinic in 2009 and published in the *Journal of Gastroenterology* (a comparison between results from samples of 3000 air force men from the 1940s and two recently collected samples) showed that the incidence of celiac disease has gone up 4.5 times. According to Dr Joseph Murray, the Mayo Clinic gastroenterologist who led the study, celiac disease is unusual but no longer rare. 'Something has changed in our environment to make it much more common,' he says, adding that these findings highlight the need to raise awareness about the increased prevalence of celiac disease and wheat-related disorders, along with higher mortality.

Another study of 10,000 persons over a duration of fifty years found that the prevalence of celiac disease had increased by 400 per cent over that period.[1]

Case for Mass Screening

Until recently, the standard approach to finding celiac disease had been to wait for people to complain of gastrointestinal symptoms and to come to the doctor for investigation. But the fact is that the number of people who do not have obvious gastrointestinal symptoms is much more (nearly eight times more). And this isn't limited to celiac. In a study of NCWS in over thirty-five Italian centres, 53 per cent of the patients had non-abdominal complaints, the most frequent being fatigue, general weakness, headaches, anxiety, foggy mind and numbness in the extremities. Anaemia, joint/muscle pain, rashes and weight loss were also symptoms. This study suggests that we may need to consider looking for celiac disease in the general population, more as we do in testing for cholesterol or blood pressure.

What Celiac Disease Teaches Us

There is a tenfold risk of other autoimmune disorders among those with celiac disease (which is accompanied by malabsorption and nutritional deficiencies). This indicates the role of micronutrients—ferritin, vitamin B12, selenium, magnesium, vitamin A, vitamin D, zinc, omega-3, to name a few—in the development of autoimmune disorders.

The increased incidence of celiac disease and the much higher risk of developing more serious autoimmune disorders reveals how important malnutrition and malabsorption are to a host body. Yet, malnutrition is often thought of as a problem of hunger and food insecurity; it is so much more than that! It is a multifaceted issue with several underlying socioeconomic factors. There is a need to build awareness, spark conversations and change attitudes about nutrition and food systems.

This heat of frustration and resentment among people is like inflammation in a host body, triggered by an extreme shortage of micronutrients in our cells (called micronutrient malnutrition).

How does the immune system react to micronutrient deficiency? By destroying healthy cells to unlock the reserves. Cells store ferritin, magnesium, vitamin B12, selenium and other critical nutrients. This abnormal activity leads to inflammation and the development of autoimmune disorders and diseases.

This is also the reason why many people's blood reports have unexplained high levels of ferritin, magnesium or vitamin B12—even when they are actually suffering from gross malnutrition and deficiencies of these elements at the cellular level.

This kind of breakdown can also happen during pregnancy, when a deficiency forces cellular breakdown to draw nutrients to the foetus—at the expense of the mother. Post-pregnancy risk of developing autoimmune disorders is documented. All this can be explained by leaky gut, malabsorption and increased demands by the body.

When there is oxygen depletion in cells, it can lead to DNA damage and abnormal cell division. The cells use anaerobic pathways to convert sugar to energy, leading to the production of lactic acid. This can be a marker to identify the presence of cancer cells (see the Warburg Effect in Chapter V).

It's very important that doctors and medical professionals understand this evidence of how essential micronutrients are. And that they become aware of the need to increase intake to benefit the patient's body.

NCWS: New Kid on the Block

Celiac disease is not the only wheat-related disease: non-celiac wheat sensitivity or NCWS is now being recognized by healthcare practitioners. Although both sets of sufferers respond to a gluten-free diet, it's important to understand the difference between NCWS and celiac disease.

NCWS may develop at any age, despite a person having consumed gluten-containing products all their life. But once a person develops this condition, they cannot tolerate gluten and experience symptoms similar to celiac disease. What they lack are the same antibodies and intestinal damage (atrophy of the villi) seen in celiac disease. Research suggests that NCWS is an innate immune response, as opposed to an autoimmune or allergic reaction.

Symptoms: Individuals with NCWS may also have a high prevalence of extra-intestinal or non-gastrointestinal symptoms such as headaches, foggy mind, joint pain and numbness in the legs, arms or fingers. Symptoms typically may appear hours or days after gluten has been ingested (they can manifest even up to seven days later). Damage with antibodies release can last up to six months even if the symptoms disappear.

NCWS is also characterized by increased intestinal permeability, but not by damaged villi as in celiac disease; this permits toxins, bacteria and undigested food proteins to seep through the gastrointestinal barrier and into the bloodstream. Research suggests that it is an early biological change that comes before the onset of several autoimmune diseases. Difficulty in losing or gaining weight are two sides of the NCWS spectrum.

Simply put, individuals with NCWS will not test positive for celiac disease in blood tests, nor do they have the same type of intestinal damage found in individuals with celiac disease. The word of caution is to seek professional help, if in doubt. Do not self-diagnose and simply going off gluten can lead to a missed diagnosis of more serious celiac disease. Although gluten-free diets are gaining popularity and are needed in celiac disease, NCWS and some other conditions, they must not become a fad.

Is GFD the New Diet Fad?

In celiac disease, adopting a gluten-free diet (GFD) is the only treatment. Elimination of gluten-containing foods also means the withdrawal of barley, rye and oats, as well as other products that contain wheat components (soy sauce, for example).

GFD should not be adopted without testing. Without professional planning and supervision, nutritional deficiencies can result from an unplanned diet and can lead to morbidity, toxicity or even mental health issues. Part of the reason is that substitutes of wheat are usually starchy and low in nutrients and partly the feeling of deprivation can trigger mood instability.

However, GFD has become so fashionable (nearly a third of Americans say they have tried GFD) that it's in real danger of reaching faddish proportions.

It is true that metabolic syndrome, allergies, cancer and autoimmune disorders have increased; it's also true that all these diseases and disorders have inflammation as the underlying cause. And this inflammation is caused by dysbiosis in the gut microbiota. We need our gut microbes to function properly—and for that, our diet needs to be healthy and balanced.

GFD is one way to achieve a better balance. It should be undertaken only after proper testing for food sensitivities. And such a diet needs to be carefully monitored for any deficiencies and calibrated to address them.

In other words, GFD is only one way and should be adopted only when it is needed. If not necessary, withdrawal of dietary gluten can result in deficiencies, as many commercially available gluten-free products have lower nutritional values. They are often deficient in fibre, folates, iron, potassium and zinc while being higher in carbohydrates, sugar and FODMAP (see Chapter V for more on FODMAPs) content. They can also be higher on the glycaemic index and glycaemic load, which can be counterproductive by increasing girth.

A study of ten healthy people without gluten sensitivity or celiac disease found that a GFD created a pro-inflammatory environment in the gut; it reduced the probiotics and thereby starved the good gut microbes that fed off them.

GFD can also result in increased toxicity from overconsumption of products like fish (which can have high levels of heavy metals like lead, arsenic and mercury). Another source of toxic compounds are the enzymes used as food additives in some commercially manufactured gluten-free foods. It is important, therefore, to avoid the potentially harmful effects of transitioning to a GFD—by personalizing the nutritional plan under the care of a professional.

Restricting or eliminating gluten should not be the only goal; the idea is to move to healthier alternatives that avoid nutritional deficiencies, toxicities or pro-inflammatory food products. Natural supplements can be added to address potential deficiencies and fortified foods, fruits and vegetables need to be increased in quantity. One diet that offers good alternatives is the elements of the Mediterranean diet (see more in Chapter X). It is rich in fibre, antioxidants, anti-inflammatory components, vitamins, trace elements, minerals, beneficial fatty acids, quality proteins and bone-building compounds. It is also metabolically balanced and affects the gut microbiome favourably.

Consulting a qualified nutrition professional who understands how the 4-G connectivity works helps to join the dots and create your very own, customized diet plan. But if you need a GFD, then it's important you **DO NOT** cheat and even occasionally eat gluten-containing foods.

Fact: People who are sensitive to gluten can often experience as much inflammation as someone with celiac disease. Therefore, cheating with gluten is not an option.

EMBRACING A WHEAT-FREE
LIFESTYLE . . . SOME FAQS

1. How do I know if I should get tested for a food sensitivity?
2. Who needs a gluten-free diet?
   a) Signs and symptoms
   b) Chronic disease including autoimmune disorders
   c) History of frequent or long-term medication
   d) First-degree relatives of celiacs
3. What are the tests that I should do?
4. What if my tests are negative?
5. Why is wheat a problem, when it is an ancient grain?
6. How should I navigate eating out?
7. Can I cheat occasionally?
8. What if there is accidental exposure or contamination?
9. Can a wheat and dairy-free diet be nutritionally adequate?
10. How do I meet my calcium levels?

Chapter V

Glucose: The Dark Side

Don't sugarcoat it

Glucose is the major fuel that powers the body's functioning. But our bodies get glucose from a vast number of sources, not just pure sugar sources such as table sugar, honey, maple syrup or agave. Glucose is the end product of ALL the carbohydrates we eat, which include fruits, breakfast cereals, biscuits, cakes, sweets, desserts and sweetened beverages, as well as staple cereals, pulses and starchy vegetables—plus the hidden sugars in processed sauces and dressings.

The indirect sources (wheat, rice and other staple cereals) are, quite literally, only one step away from glucose: it may surprise you that **one slice of bread is equal to a tablespoon of sugar.**

Black Effect

White sugar has a dark effect on us: when we add sugar to our tea and coffee, we are simply adding extra calories, calories that have zero nutrients—except that we like the taste. Worse, sugars in the form of candy, pastries or ice cream are calorie-heavy and nutrient-light. It's important to realize that although we believe that sugars boost energy levels, the reverse is true: an excess of sugar depletes energy levels by causing an imbalance in insulin and hypoglycemia. Insulin is the hormone that regulates sugar in the body.

Until recently, the role of sugar management was considered important only for those who were managing diabetes or were at risk of developing it. However, any diet loaded with sugars and refined carbohydrates promotes insulin resistance. It is a condition in which cells are unable to fully utilize sugars from the blood, causing the pancreas to produce more insulin, until it can no longer keep pace with the demand. That leads to increased girth and hence visceral fat, inflammation, metabolic syndrome, pre-diabetes, Type 2 diabetes and/or cardiovascular disease.

Obesity and Sugar Intake

We associate celebrations with desserts, cakes, halwa, etc., and so sugar cannot just be done away with. But remember the equation: just one teaspoon of sugar in your daily tea or coffee can result in a gain of 1 kg of body fat per year and trigger insulin resistance and a large girth.

Diabetes/Sugar and Insulin Resistance

A study conducted in 2016 by IPSOS (a global leader in market research) across countries on sugar consumption found that over 50 per cent of Indian respondents reported consuming more than the permissible limit (twelve teaspoons a day, across all forms). India is the diabetes capital of the world, with 49 per cent of the world's diabetics, putting an enormous health burden on strained resources.

Conventional wisdom is that Type 2 diabetes results from obesity—it is true that obesity does push the host body towards insulin resistance (hormonal imbalance) and that obesity is accelerated among those people with a family history of Type 2 diabetes. But recent studies show that in India, 20 to 30 per cent of diabetics are not obese. They are quite thin, in fact.

This is not exactly a dichotomy: the study found that even those Indians who were not obese (had a BMI [Body Mass Index] of 25 or less) or even thin (a BMI of under 19) actually had a high proportion of abdominal fat and low muscle mass. And they tended to have fatty livers and pancreas, which contributed to insulin resistance.

Insulin is a body-building hormone that preferentially increases girth around the abdomen. Insulin resistance means that the body doesn't allow the hormone insulin to supply sugar to the cells; so blood sugar levels are elevated while the cells are starving. The signal thus sent to the pancreas is to produce more insulin and so on. Excess insulin in the blood increases inflammation and can eventually lead to Type 2 diabetes.

Insulin resistance can lead not just to diabetes but to abnormal cholesterol levels—and of the bad kind. It increases triglycerides and LDL and lowers HDL— the good cholesterol. It can also cause high levels of uric acid, fatty liver and an imbalance of reproductive hormones (leading to PCOS) as well as contribute to high blood pressure. These can also impact the skin adversely. Conditions like acne, alopecia, dandruff, eczema and psoriasis are associated with high insulin levels in the blood and inflammation.

While insulin resistance and diabetes are not directly correlated to excess intake of sugar, either as sugar, sweets or carbohydrates, the extra consumption does lead to accumulation of abdominal or visceral fat—and that is deeply connected to the development of insulin resistance, internal inflammation and other diseases.

Red Flags of Insulin Imbalance or Unstable Blood Sugar

- Intense cravings for sugar
- Need to eat frequently (every two hours) or right after a meal
- Headaches if there are long gaps between meals
- Need frequent pick-me-ups like coffee and tea throughout the day
- Irritability, lightheadedness, shakiness or weakness or fatigue with long gaps between meals

Glucose and Cancer

As long ago as the 1930s, Dr Otto Warburg's research into the metabolism of cancerous tumours and examination of cancer cells found that they thrive in a low-oxygen, low-alkaline environment. And that in such a situation, cancerous cells were able to rely on glucose fermentation rather than respiration (which uses oxygen) to produce energy and grow. Cancer cells are able to use glucose even in the absence of oxygen. This is called the Warburg Effect.

Gut Health

If this wasn't enough, a diet rich in refined sugar and processed foods can change the microbial balance in the gut; it significantly decreases the number of good bacteria. This can lead to dysbiosis and bloating and may worsen gastrointestinal complaints like flatulence and acidity. High amounts of refined sugars lead to chronic inflammation. A condition called candidiasis is an overgrowth of a yeast fungus, encouraged by sugar. Candidiasis can create an infection in the mouth, throat, vagina or gut. It is worsened by other toxins, such as pesticides, excessive processed food, refined flours, alcohol and dairy products in the gut, leading to a leaky gut.

Sugar and Immunity

Abnormal gut flora can also lower immunity and cause allergies, skin problems like acne, eczema, psoriasis and nutritional deficiencies (B vitamins, zinc, chromium and other vital nutrients).

Where Is Sugar Hiding?

The problem with sugar isn't just avoiding the obvious sugar one adds or consumes in desserts; there are concealed sugars lurking in many foods that we could be unaware of.

Sugar hides in many places. It's insidiously present in soft drinks and sharbats, both traditional ones and carbonated beverages. Manufacturers use different names for added sugars in order to hide the fact of their presence: high-fructose corn syrup, maltose, dextrose, maltodextrin and the like.

Honey, jaggery, maple syrup and cane syrup are natural forms and eventually break down as glucose in the body but are equally loaded with sugar. The effect of all these is to add to the total consumption burden on the body.

Then there are short-chain sugars that are hard to digest (FODMAPs), which can cause a wide range of gastrointestinal symptoms in those who are sensitive to them.

FODMAP: An Acronym to Avoid

Researchers at Monash University in Melbourne coined the term 'FODMAP'—a simple acronym for the convoluted Fermentable oligo-, di-, and mono-saccharides and polyols. These are a group of poorly absorbed short-chain carbohydrates (sugars) that are resistant to digestion. Instead of being absorbed into the bloodstream via the normal digestive process, they reach the colon in an undigested state.

In most people, the majority of the FODMAPs pass out undigested, like fibre. In fact, dietary fibre feeds good gut bacteria and produces methane, which is normal. But the process of metabolism of food produces acids and since the body needs to maintain its pH or acid–alkali balance (the pH needs to be slightly tilted towards alkaline), it pulls alkalinity to restore equilibrium. This is a delicate equation and if there are undigested foods present, they can ferment.

In people who are sensitive to FODMAPs, they ferment, and the bacteria then using them as fuel are unfriendly and produce hydrogen, which can lead to stomach cramps, constipation and bloating. Worse, they can draw liquid into the colon and cause diarrhoea and inflammation.

FODMAPs Deconstructed

Fermentable refers to the process through which gut bacteria break down undigested carbohydrates to produce gases (hydrogen, methane and carbon dioxide). **Oligosaccharides** include fructooligosaccharides (fructans) and galactooligosaccharides (galactans). Fructans are found in wheat, rye, onions and garlic. Wheat and wheat products such as pasta, bread, cereals, crackers and biscuits are a major source of fructans. Galactans are found in legumes and pulses such as chickpeas, beans and lentils.

Disaccharides are carbohydrates that include two units of monosaccharides, such as sucrose, which, with glucose and fructose, forms table sugar, and lactose, which is formed when galactose combines with glucose. **Monosaccharides** are the most basic carbohydrates and include galactose (a single, molecular form of sugar found in milk, yogurt, cheese and other dairy products, as is lactose) and fructose or fruit sugar, found not only in fruit but in honey, apples and high-fructose corn syrup (an ingredient of many sauces, salad dressings, sweet yogurt, canned fruit, etc.). However, the levels of fructose in fruit differ considerably: apples and watermelon, for instance, contain much more and bananas and blueberries less. **(A) and (P) Polyols** are sugar alcohols such as sorbitol, mannitol and xylitol. They are found in some fruits and vegetables and are used as artificial sweeteners in sugar-free mints/gums.

The low FODMAP food plan is a relatively new approach to managing gastrointestinal disorders and is gaining recognition as an effective diet for managing irritable bowel syndrome (IBS), inflammatory bowel diseases such as Crohn's or ulcerative colitis, bloating or flatulence. It also helps reduce symptoms in people who have FIGD—functional gastrointestinal disorders—a term that covers a range of digestive issues. The aim is to identify which FODMAP foods, if any, cause symptoms. It involves restricting certain foods for up to six to eight weeks and then re-introducing them systematically back into the diet through 'food challenges' to identify any trigger foods.

Remember, a low FODMAP plan is not a 'No-FODMAP plan', as some foods contain FODMAPS that act like prebiotic fibre and help friendly gut bacteria to function properly. But if you frequently experience digestive issues, FODMAPs could be right at the top of the list of suspects.

Nor is this a 'lifetime' diet. After the restrictive period is over, most people can resume their usual diet—with a few high-FODMAP foods to be avoided or consumed in small quantities. A review in the journal *Nutrition in Clinical Practice* in 2013 reported that nearly 86 per cent of patients with IBS achieved relief in overall gastrointestinal symptoms and, more specifically, bloating, flatulence, abdominal pain and altered bowel habits after following a low FODMAP diet.

HIGH FODMAP FOODS

- Most dairy
- Sweeteners
- Dressings and sauces with HFCS
- Fruits such as watermelon, apricots, cherries, dates, figs, pears
- Canned fruit
- Legumes such as rajma, chickpeas, lentils
- Vegetables such as broccoli, beetroot, cauliflower, garlic, mushrooms, onions, okra, peas and asparagus
- Beer, soft drinks, fruit juice and soy milk

LOW FODMAP FOODS

- Fish and eggs
- Fats and oils
- Nuts, except pistachios
- Most other fruits
- Lactose-free dairy products
- Hard cheeses such as Parmesan, and soft, aged ones such as Camembert
- Gluten-free cereals such as millets or rice
- Tea and coffee

Tips for a low FODMAP Diet

Avoid high FODMAP foods for six weeks. After this, add high FODMAP foods one at a time back into your diet in small amounts, to identify which of them could be the 'trigger' to your symptoms.

Limit the foods that activate your particular symptoms.

Read food labels carefully when you shop. Avoid foods made with high FODMAPs such as HFCS, honey, wheat and soy. However, a food could be an overall low FODMAP food if a high FODMAP food is listed as the last ingredient.

Buy gluten-free grains. However, you do not need to follow a 100 per cent gluten-free diet as the focus is on FODMAPs, not gluten. Look for gluten-free grains made with low FODMAPs, such as potato, quinoa, rice or corn.

But, before you embark on food planning that eliminates any categories of food from your nutrition regime, it's advisable to consult a healthcare professional—this should **NOT** be undertaken without monitoring. Otherwise, you might be too unnecessarily restrictive; for instance, there are some tests that can tell whether you need to avoid lactose or fructose. Also, you might eliminate some food that is useful, if not essential, to other requirements of the body.

Sugar High—and Low

Most of the time, the sugar we invariably consume is not gur or jaggery, but the most refined form—white sugar—and this is highly addictive. The reason is simple: when we eat sugar, a neurotransmitter called dopamine is released. That means that we get a pleasure high, just as with certain drugs. And it also has exactly the same diminishing marginal benefit as drugs do—as we eat more of the sugar, the brain adjusts by releasing less dopamine each time, so we need more and more to get the same high. That is addiction.

Your Sugar Cravings Are Not about Willpower!

Sugar is highly addictive. In fact, as a Connecticut College study in 2013, published in *Science News*,[1] found, cookies can fire more neurons in the brain's pleasure centre in rats than cocaine does. Another Princeton study found that rats developed addictive behaviour—craving, bingeing and withdrawal—to sugar. Cassie Bjork, founder of HealthySimpleLife. com points out that sugar is more addictive than cocaine, saying, 'Sugar activates the opiate receptors in our brain and affects the reward centre, which leads to compulsive behaviour, despite the negative consequences like weight gain, headaches, hormonal imbalances and more.'

The WHO considers reducing daily sugar intake to half, from 10 per cent to 5 per cent of the total caloric intake, which is about four to six teaspoons a day for an average 2000 calories a day diet.[2]

Remember the fact that 'stressed' when spelt backwards is—desserts.

Chapter VI

Girth: Figure It Out

The direct correlation between obesity and an increased risk of developing cardiac disease, diabetes or stroke is well known. But what we are seeing today is a growing number of relatively thin or slim people with the same disorders that have been historically linked to extra weight. These include diabetes, high blood pressure, arthritis, fatty liver, varicose veins and gout. Polycystic ovarian syndrome, gestational diabetes and pregnancy-related complications are becoming more and more common in slim people.

So, What Is the Reason?

The reason is simple: while being overweight is an indicator of underlying health issues, it is **not** the only indicator of ill health. As mentioned in Chapter II, 'The 4-G Connectivity', body fat is not as important as **where** this body fat is distributed. That's because fat behaves differently in the body, depending on its location. An overall slim person who carries excess weight on the belly is far more vulnerable to inflammatory diseases than someone who has fat thighs and legs. These are the thin–fat people, with normal posterior bodies but a bulge on the belly.

Subcutaneous fat is fat which is just under the skin. Visceral fat, on the other hand, the fat that is deposited around the internal organs (the liver, kidneys and intestines) is the dangerous one, with serious health implications.

Relevance of Girth

Interestingly, even though individuals may not have digestive issues, they may have a leaky gut indicated by high zonulin levels—a marker of leaky gut. Higher zonulin levels are associated with higher waist circumference as well as higher blood pressure and fasting glucose levels. Clearly, higher zonulin levels and leaky gut are associated with visceral fat and an increased risk of inflammatory diseases.[1]

There are several indices that help determine the location of body fat. Waist circumference is an important measure of the distribution of fat. It's important, however, that when measuring the waist, one must measure the maximum part. A waist circumference of less than 31.5 inches (80 cm) in women and 35.5 inches (90 cm) in men is considered acceptable for Indian women and men, respectively.

A more recent tool to measure is the waist-to-height ratio; it's considered more accurate in measuring levels of visceral fat. Ideally, the waist should be half the height. Another tool using bio-impedance is simple body composition analysis.

And one really good gauge of the kind of fat we have is a simple one—check your shape in a mirror!

Contour Counts

The apple shape, also known as male pattern, central or trunk obesity, is the visceral kind of fat and is associated with inflammation and insulin resistance, and a wide range of diseases. The pear shape, or female pattern obesity, is fat around the hips and thighs, and is less likely to be associated with disease. It's the muffin tops, the roll of fat around the abdomen, the beer belly, that is the kind of fat that substantially increases the risk of developing diseases.

Today, however, from the beer belly, it has transformed into the wheat belly!

What is causing us to lose the battle of the bulge? It's the connection between gluten, glucose (sugars) in the diet, and their adverse impact on gut health that results in the wheat belly. And the overall effect of adding girth (central mass obesity) to the other three Gs is the quadruple health whammy.

Of course, if you have central obesity or girth, high insulin levels (also known as insulin resistance) may eventually catch up as increased overall body weight and increased BMI.

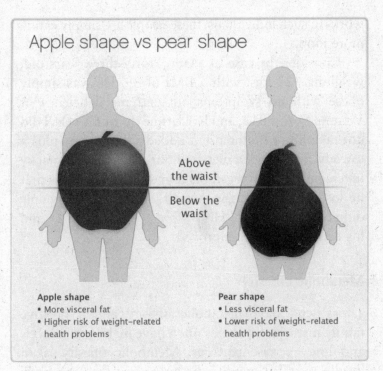

Fig. 3

Simple Obesity

In my previous book, *The Diet Doctor*, I referred to simple and metabolic obesity as two entities. The former is the type in which a person gains overall weight, possibly in several typical areas, such as arms, thighs, legs, abdomen and hips. There is usually no family history of diabetes or insulin resistance. Such people gain weight and lose it relatively easily. They find it easy to gain weight, but weight loss from reducing calories is also quick. The calories in and calories out equation works in such individuals; these people are simply eating more food.

Consider the case of Manoj, forty-three years old, weighing 122 kgs, with a BMI of 39. He was simply obese with no symptoms but extreme deficiency of Vitamin D and B12, and borderline thyroid levels. I did not take him off gluten but added supplements plus a low glycaemic index diet—a filling breakfast, a snacky lunch and an only vegetable dinner. The result was that he lost 45 kgs in eight months, so much that people didn't recognize him! His BMI also dropped to 24 and his deficiencies also improved.

Metabolic Obesity

Those who have metabolic obesity and a positive family history of diabetes often have high insulin levels and low exercise patterns. Metabolic obesity is an insulin-resistant condition; this means that the body doesn't respond to insulin in a normal manner. That's because some of the insulin receptor cells have become ineffective. The pancreas, therefore, needs to produce more insulin to regulate blood sugar. So, a person with metabolic obesity produces higher levels of insulin to metabolize the same amount of sugar consumed than someone with simple obesity.

Insulin levels have a direct and proportionate effect on the storage of fat by the body, particularly in the visceral organs such as the liver, gall bladder, pancreas and spleen. Those with metabolic obesity, therefore, are more prone to ill health and find it more difficult to lose the fat. Such people respond better to a low carbohydrate diet and increased exercise as we did with Mr Singh, a forty-seven-year-old corporate executive, 5 ft 7 inches tall, weighing 119 kgs. His waist measurement was 51 inches and his BMI was 40. He also had symptoms of alopecia (baldness), dark thickened skin in the armpits (*acanthosis nigricans*), warts and skin tags, and suffered from sleep apnea (snoring) and insulin resistance. He had massive sugar cravings—on average, he would consume half a kilo of sweets a day!

The symptoms might have seemed varied, but the diagnosis was singular: this was a case of metabolic obesity. His c-reactive protein (a marker of inflammation) was high at 4.07, thyroid borderline and he had low vitamin B12 and D3 levels. Without vastly reducing his caloric intake, we simply altered **what** he was eating. His breakfast would typically be cornflakes and milk, plus the massive sweets; this was substituted by eggs and cheelas. For lunch, he used to have three rotis; we suggested salad and sprouts. Similarly, for dinner, inflammatory grains were substituted by healthier alternatives, and proteins and vegetables were added.

The results were that within a month, the snoring was gone and his sugar craving was history. His thyroid and inflammation levels corrected themselves and in five months, he had reached 86 kg, a huge weight loss of 33 kg! His waist dropped to 37 inches and he got bitten by the fitness bug; he began exercising regularly. He was one of the clinic's biggest (weight) losers, but a winner in the health stakes!

Obesity of the Third Kind

Now, I would like to add a third type of obesity, called Immunogenic Obesity. When there is a failure to respond to a reduction in carbohydrates and calories, and increased exercise, it is time to look deeper into the functioning of the gut. This form of obesity, which I call immunogenic obesity, according to the latest research, is rooted in the functioning of the gut microbiome (see more in Chapter I, 'The Gut Matters'). This kind of obesity is caused by imbalanced gut flora, and the immune system reacting to foods that we are sensitive to, most common among them being gluten, some other grains and/or dairy. In fact, in my clinical experience, immunogenic obesity is what leads to metabolic obesity and it is highly inflammatory.

Immunogenic obesity develops when there is an adverse effect on the gut. It is a condition that is a precursor to serious autoimmune disorders and even malignancy; it increases the risk of developing colon, prostate, endometrial and colon cancer, and significantly increases the chances of breast cancer in postmenopausal women.

For the past decade or more, most of my patients are struggling and are unable to lose weight even though they are eating as little or even fewer than 1000 calories and working out for anything between one and two hours. These individuals eat barely one chapati in every meal or not even that at times.

Many are consuming superfoods and supplements too. Just eliminating wheat and certain grains, and substituting them with selected grains, the process of losing weight begins and the bloating disappears. Interestingly, many of such cases come with symptoms of fatigue, nutritional deficiencies, such as vitamin D and B12, and autoimmune disorders, skin or hair problems, hormonal imbalances or mental health issues. With dietary corrections, they not only achieve weight loss but also resolve their health issues. Clearly, this form of obesity is not driven by calories but by the inflammation of the immune system.

Gut Microbiome and Weight

How does the gut microbiome influence weight gain? Recent studies showed that the trillions of bacteria that reside in the gut can affect weight. For instance, in some studies, when bacteria from obese mice were injected into lean mice and vice versa, they gained weight. A leaky gut, too, can be connected to insulin resistance and obesity because when it becomes permeable, factors such as bacterial imbalance, a poor diet or an imbalanced one can lead to obesity.

Obese and Disease

I'm fat and I'm happy! Do you hear this often? It's not true, however. Being overweight is not a happy feeling for the body. We are designed to be lean and full of energy. Carrying extra weight does nothing to improve energy levels.

The reverse is true: for every extra kg over an optimal weight, your body feels more sluggish and has to work harder to accomplish the same daily activities. For every gain over one's ideal body weight, the risks don't just add up, they multiply. It worsens the quality of life in every way; often, it also lowers the quantity of life.

As it happened with a male patient who came to us. He was forty-three years old, weighed 116 kg and had a BMI of 41. Surprisingly, he was not a big eater but had added weight disproportionate to the calories consumed.

Losing weight was very challenging for him as he had developed hypothyroidism at age thirty. He had pain in his back and legs, a problem breathing and severe alopecia. His food tolerance tests showed reactions to gluten and dairy. So he was taken off gluten, dairy, corn and soya. He was given controlled grains and supplements for deficiencies. Additionally, we added gut-healing preparations to his diet. Within a month, his glucose levels normalized and his pain and breathlessness subsided. In one year, his weight dropped to 90 kg.

Obesity doesn't just burden the individual; it also imposes a heavy monetary cost on overall health services. A 2005 International Labour Organization (ILO) study estimated that poor diets cost up to 20 per cent in loss of productivity, either due to malnutrition in developing countries or excess weight and obesity in developed economies.[1]

So What Should You Weigh?

It's not the same for everyone. And how much excess weight you might have is only part of the problem;

how the fat is distributed is more important. Weight-watching is not just about reaching a particular weight goal. The aim is to feel fit and fine. There are established indicators to help determine YOUR ideal body weight, how the fat in your body is distributed and what your body shape is.

These need to be worked out in tandem to measure accurately what your weight and body composition should be.

BMI Km/m^2	Risk of Disease Waist—Men: under 102 cm Women: less than 88 cm	Risk of Disease Men: over 102 cm Women: over 88 cm
Underweight: less than 18		
Normal 18.5–24.9		
Overweight 25–29.9	Increased	High
Obesity I 30.0–35.9	High	Very high
Obesity II 35.0–35.9	Very high	Very high
Obesity III more than 40	Extremely high	Extremely high
(Source: Data from WHO on managing obesity)		

Chapter VII

The P Factors: Thirty-Five Leads to a Leaky Gut

'People are fed by the food industry, which pays no attention to health; and are treated by the health industry, which pays no attention to food'
—Wellness expert Dr Mark Hyman

Apart from the interaction between the four Gs, there are a number of **other factors** that affect the protective barrier of our gut and intestinal permeability. Some work for us and others militate against our good health (and should be controlled). We need to understand and apply this knowledge in the clearest manner possible to maintain good gut balance and stay healthy. I call these the '35 Ps'; they track a path of information that you can use to power up your gut microbiome and make it work for you rather than against you, and rebuild the broken barrier of a leaky gut.

Dietary

1. **Protein Sensitivity, Food Intolerances and Allergies, and Adverse Reactions to Food:** As mentioned in Chapter III, as much as a third of the world's population is estimated to be sensitive to gluten, the protein in wheat. This sensitivity can lead to a leaky gut and sets the stage for other food intolerances or allergies. These can be reactions to soya, corn, oats, eggs and even buckwheat and nuts, to name a few common ones.

   Milk too contains proteins such as casein, which can cause abnormal reactions. This is because it has a similarity to gluten and our immune system treats it the same. When the body reacts to these proteins, it causes inflammation, dysbiosis and eventually permeability (leaky gut).

   Just as in the case of wheat gluten, antibodies to these proteins can potentially cause symptoms inside the gut (bloating, hyperacidity, reflux, constipation, etc.) or outside the gut (rashes, skin conditions, hair issues, joint pains, asthma and other respiratory issues, depression and anxiety). About 50 per cent of gluten-intolerant people are also dairy-intolerant, but this should not be confused with lactose intolerance, which is an intolerance to milk sugar.

2. **Poor Nutrition and Deficiencies:** Dietary nutrients can affect the gut microbiome. It's essential to provide beneficial nutrients for gut health, maintain gut integrity and prevent a leaky gut. Inadequate

food intake, poor appetite, or eating food of poor quality (highly processed, refined foods that are calorie-heavy but nutritionally light) is a two-way relationship—poor nutritional status is linked to a leaky gut and the other way around too. A leaky gut can compromise the absorption of nutrients.

This malabsorption and resultant deficiencies can trigger the autoimmunity switch. Essential nutrients whose deficiency is associated with autoimmunity are vitamin A (which calms the immune system), vitamin D (which lowers inflammation and boosts immunity), iron, magnesium, zinc and selenium, to name a few.

3. **Processed and Junk Food:** A diet rich in processed or junk food leads to a change in the gut microbiome and a leaky gut, on two accounts: a) because of low-nutrient and low-fibre intake and b) because of unhealthy additives and chemical preservatives present in such foods. In addition, they are laced with poor-quality fats and trans-fatty acids, which are known to increase inflammation. High sugar content in such foods also disturbs the gut microbiome. Such foods are associated with increased inflammation, poor immunity, and higher rates of cancer and autoimmune diseases. Evidence shows that these diets lead to deficiencies of vitamin D, iron, zinc and more.

Animal protein like chicken, for instance, is often injected with hormones, antibiotics or vaccines to ensure growth and yield. Chicks (35–40 gm) are grown to 2–2.5 kg in thirty-five to forty days with the help of such injections. The same is true of milk production (injecting cows to achieve higher milk yield). Ingesting these products is sure to impact the gut microbiome adversely.

4. **Portions and Too Much Food:** Eating too much leads to obesity, which shifts the microbiome negatively. And if our portions contain addictive components such as gluten and sugar, the need to keep eating more of the same increases exponentially. Gut microbiome disturbance can both alter eating behaviour and get impacted by large portions. Eating disorders can be traced to dysbiosis and both are linked to compromised gut integrity.

5. **The PM Factor (Eating Late and Post-Work Chaos):** Research from the University of Chicago[2] highlights that the millions of microbes that live in the intestines respond to altered sleep, waking and feeding schedules of the host. 'If the host is eating at the wrong time, the microbes can adapt to that, but it throws off their timing,' says Vanessa Leon, the University of Chicago researcher who led the study.

6. **Poor Sleep Patterns:** Sleep is the body's pause button. Sleep quality again is a two-way relationship: poor sleep (an inadequate number of hours or poor quality) alters gut function and vice versa. In both cases, the effect on the gut microbiome is intimately connected with the development of dysbiosis and leaky gut. The University of Chicago's study, cited in the previous

point, found that model tissue, when exposed to intestinal tissue from sleep-disturbed mice, proved to be leaky while that from rested mice was not.

7. *Praana* or 'Live' Food: This is food which is loaded with enzymes. Enzymes are protein-rich substances that support the functions of the body, as they are catalysts in the chemical reactions that occur internally. Breathing, digestion and even the functioning of the heart are all functions that depend on enzymes.

   The gut microbiome gets boosted by food rich in enzymes. All fresh vegetables, fruits and fermented and sprouted foods provide enzymes and impact gut integrity positively. Inadequate intake of these can impair the gut and contribute to the development of a leaky gut.

8. **Preservatives, Artificial Colours and Sweeteners**: Research on the effect of preservatives on health is limited but there is little doubt that the impact on gut flora balance is adverse. Sulfites, among the most common preservatives, limit the growth of beneficial gut bacteria such as Lactobacillus and S. thermophilus, among others. In a study conducted at Georgia State University and published in 2015 in *Nature*, emulsifiers, an artificial preservative used in many processed foods such as ice creams and mayonnaise, altered the make-up of bacteria in the colon and the bacteria developed glucose intolerance and obesity.

   Another source of harmful compounds are enzymes used as additives in a variety of processed food products, including many that are gluten-free. Microbial transglutaminase (mTG) is one such; it's mostly not labelled and its use is hidden. It's used to bind proteins (it is also called 'meat glue') and it changes both the physical properties and immunogenic nature of many gluten-free products. Since it mimics the manner in which tissue transglutaminase (tTG—an enzyme that fixes damage in the body and is an indicator of celiac disease) functions, it can modify gliadin peptides by cross-linking them, which encourages intolerance of gluten.

mTG has been classified as 'safe' in the US, but the European Union banned its use in food products in 2018. Its presence in gluten-free products means that for those adopting a gluten-free diet, fresh alternative grains rather than processed products should be the choice for their plate.

9. **Protein and Other Supplements**: They are called health supplements, but they don't always contribute positively to the gut and thereby, health. Most avid exercise-oriented people are asked to take protein supplements by their coaches. While those who undertake endurance training might well require an increased amount of protein in their diets, there are plenty of protein sources available in natural food. The addition of supplements is warranted only in certain conditions. Excess animal protein can also create an acidic environment in the body, which is counterproductive and increases inflammation.

Whey and soya protein are the stars of the supplementary universe because they are a rich source of essential amino acids. But in those with a sensitivity to dairy or gluten, these will have a negative effect because of the undesirable impact on the gut.

10. *Paani* (**Water**) **and Fluid Intake**: Dehydration or less water in the body can lead to an inflammatory situation. Good mucosal (lining) hydration is necessary for normal protective intestinal barrier function. A compromised barrier function is certainly a prelude to a leaky gut. Keeping your body well-hydrated is essential—the body is 70 per cent water.

11. **Pick-Me-Ups** (**Tea and Coffee**): There is a large body of evidence[1] with respect to green tea; up to four or five cups daily are reported to increase the healthy bifidobacterium. Even black tea has been reported to modulate a favourable shift in the ratio of firmicutes to bacteroidetes (fat-storage to fat-burning bacteria). Similar effects have been reported in small studies on coffee involving three cups daily. These studies need to be followed up, yet preliminary evidence suggests a positive effect on the diversity of gut flora and thereby gut integrity.

12. **pH** (**Alkaline/Acidic**) **Balance**: A possible effect of improvement in gut microbiota with a shift to a more alkaline diet and water has a favourable effect on the gut microbiome. This is more relevant in modern lifestyles and diets that are exposed to acidic high protein and processed foods. As much as 70 per cent of all antibiotics used in the US is

for animals (as growth enhancers) and is a cause for the rampant increase in antibiotic-resistant disease in humans.

Body chemistry is about maintaining the acid-base balance: to stay healthy, the pH of the body should be tilted to the alkaline, ideally at about 7.4. This process is controlled by the kidneys and the lungs, but the influence of nutrition is vital. All foods, when digested, leave a residue or ash, which can be acidic, alkaline or neutral. Proteins produce an acidic residue; fruits and vegetables leave an alkaline one, even if they are sour or acidic (such as lemons or oranges). A diet rich in proteins and low in vegetables can cause metabolic acidosis (when the pH falls below 7.35), inflammation and disease. Diet must, therefore, balance acidic- and alkaline-forming foods.

13. **Prebiotics and Probiotics:** The composition of the gut microbiome, if unbalanced, can lead to inflammation and a leaky gut. In order to create a better balance, what we can add to the diet are probiotics and prebiotics. Traditional knowledge has shown that a diet rich in cultured (foods with 'live' bacteria) are useful in helping maintain gut integrity. This is why there is a long tradition of using microbial cultures to ferment food, from yogurt to cheese to pickles, etc.

Probiotics are good bacteria and microbes (such as lactobacillus and bifidobacterium); they have been defined as 'live microbial food which helps the host . . . by improving its intestinal microbial balance'. Prebiotics are food for the good bacteria. The concept of prebiotics is relatively new—it was introduced by a research paper in 1995.[3] They defined prebiotics as 'a non-digestible food ingredient that beneficially affects the host by selectively stimulating the growth and/or activity of one or a limited number of bacteria in the colon'.

Both pro- and prebiotics play important roles in helping maintain gut health. Consumption of probiotics, through food and supplements, helps restore gut flora balance. In fact, their addition can help stabilize the gut's barrier function, counteract local dysfunction and prevent infectious pathogens from proliferating. Prebiotics are equally important: they are contained in those carbohydrates (read fibre) that we cannot digest but the gut-friendly bacteria can and do feed on. All foods rich in soluble fibre, including fermentable oligosaccharides (FOS) are rich in prebiotics and impact gut integrity positively.

But Gibson and Roverford, in their research paper, also introduced the concept of synbiotics, which they said were a mix of pro- and prebiotics that improve the host's gut with their content of live microbial supplements and by stimulating the growth of beneficial bacteria.[4]

Toxins and Environment

14. **Painkillers, Antibiotics and Other Drugs:** Each chemical you ingest is a blow to the gut balance.

Antibiotics are obviously the big offenders here as they kill both the good and bad microbes. There is also evidence that early childhood exposure to antibiotics can lead to several gastrointestinal, immunologic, mental health and neurological conditions.[5] It can play havoc with your gut lining and cause food sensitivities and a leaky gut.

A study[6] led by scientists at Stanford University (funded by the National Institute of Allergy and Infectious Diseases) found that when oral antibiotics kill gut microorganisms, it can alter the human response to diseases. Repeated use of antibiotics creates an imbalance in the gut microbiota, and when microbes are killed off by the trillion, the host body can find that yeast overgrowth can occur in the absence of other bacteria. Nature, as you know, hates a vacuum!

Chemotherapy too adversely affects the gut microbiota, inducing dysbiosis and altered physiological and psychological function. Medicines based on chemical ingredients can damage the diversity of microbiota and promote dysbiosis and leaky gut.

Painkillers, which people often pop without even consulting a doctor, are really a prescription for intestinal damage; over time, they can lead to inflammation in the stomach and the duodenum (the first part of the small intestine). Overuse of painkillers and anti-inflammatory drugs reduces the secretion of protective prostaglandins, which protect the gut; this makes the gut more prone to injury and increases permeability.

15. **Pesticides, Poisons, Hormones, Chemicals and GM Foods**: While the potential risk from the consumption of genetically modified transgenic crops remains a controversial subject, the effect of pesticides (such as glyphosates, as mentioned in Chapter III, and others) on dysbiosis and leaky gut is clearly established.

Much of what we eat today is treated with pesticides, as farmers are encouraged to improve yield through their use. While we perceive these as long-term poisons, the truth is that they also affect us on a daily basis, by altering our gut flora negatively. This is a precursor to developing a leaky gut and food sensitivities.

Worse, the long-term body damage pesticides can do is serious: they are cumulative poisons, so the levels increase with time; they are carcinogenic (capable of causing cancers), mutagenic (genetic mutations) and teratogenic (birth defects). They also play significant roles in increasing the incidence of reproductive disorders.

16. **Pollution, Heavy Metals (Mercury, Arsenic, Lead)**: Non-absorbed heavy metals in the environment have a direct impact on the gut microbiota and overall gut integrity. Several studies have documented this impact. In a 2014 study,[7] mice were exposed to 10ppm arsenic for four weeks. It resulted in significant changes in the intestinal flora. Lead is another heavy metal that has become a concern because of contamination of drinking water or even inhalation from old

cans of paint. Exposing mice to lead in drinking water altered the diversity of their microbiome. Exposure to such chemicals can lead to widespread disruption in the microbiome, increasing the risk of developing a leaky gut.

17. **Plastic, Endocrine Disrupters and the Pill:** Researchers in a recent study,[8] carried out by the Medical University of Vienna in Austria, have found that an average daily motion contains 200 pieces of microplastics, said lead researcher Dr Philipp Schwabl. Do the math: that's 73,000 pieces of microplastic every year, ingested through our food and drink (many of them through bottled water and some through the fish we eat). These microparticles accumulate in the gut and can absorb toxic chemicals, and the smallest particles can enter the bloodstream and the lymphatic system.

Endocrine disruptors are chemicals that can interfere with the endocrine or hormonal system. They are called xenoestrogens as many of them imitate oestrogen. Xeno means foreign, so foreign oestrogen or hormones are regarded as serious hazards to health and the ecosystem. Xenoestrogens include synthetic oestrogen (ethinylestradiol) used in the contraceptive pill consumed so extensively among women to treat hormonal disorders. Not surprising then, that women on the pill develop food sensitivities.

Other disruptors, such as PCBs (polychlorinated biphenyls), bisphenol A and phthalates, are found in household products such as plastic bottles, detergents, pesticides and even cosmetics. Heating water in plastic bottles, even by keeping them exposed to sunlight in a car, leaches phthalates. An ongoing University of California study[9] is examining how exposure to endocrine disruptors in mice and humans changes the structure of gut microbiota and triggers dysbiosis of the gut microbial community.

Glyphosates are also known endocrine disruptors and inhibit hormones, causing an imbalance in hormone levels. They also inhibit certain enzymes (like cytochrome P450) that are involved in detoxifying environmental toxins. And because they have the ability to bind to micronutrient elements like iron, copper, cobalt and other minerals, ingestion can lead to deficiencies in their levels.

18. **Poor Soils and Nutritional Status Due to Poor Agricultural Practices**: Poor nutrition can impair our gut lining. If our soils are depleted in micro-nutrients, our food will be low in them too (see Chapter XII for essential minerals), which can impact our gut integrity.

19. **Politics and Food Lobbies**: The power of food politics and policies can impact what we end up eating and the quality of what we eat. These indirectly affect our food choices; today we have sugar, grain and dairy lobbies, to name a few. And big pharma too. The biggest manufacturers of cancer drugs are also the largest producers of

pesticides. Many school programmes have been supported by junk food manufacturers. Policies are developed for larger populations and until guidelines change, which takes more than a decade, one has to take individual responsibility for making informed choices; we know that certain grains like wheat, and foods like sugar, dairy and junk food, can induce dysbiosis and a leaky gut.

Life Cycle

20. **Plain and Simple Age:** Just as our outer skin thins with age, so does our gut lining. Our gut becomes frail with age and more prone to inflammation. In a youthful gut, the cells are packed tight. As the host ages, the viability of the cells in the gut is reduced and this makes them more vulnerable to damage; the gut becomes more permeable and more prone to inflammation, and the natural repair process slows down as well. The ageing process itself involves a reduction in the host body's ability to maintain a healthy gut flora balance and therefore, develops age-related immune disturbances and metabolic dysfunction, and eventually loss of oral tolerance to certain foods like wheat and dairy. The ageing process cannot be wished away, but the loss of gut integrity can be managed with a better diet, plenty of fresh fruit and vegetables and the elimination of processed and fried foods.

21. **Placental Crossovers and Maternal Malnutrition:** The placenta plays a crucial role in pregnancy. It's a natural barrier between the mother and the foetus and provides oxygen and nutrients to the growing baby. But it can also pass on antibodies to foods, particularly in the third trimester. According to recent reports, the gut flora of a pregnant woman in the third trimester is similar to that of an individual with inflammatory bowel disease. Antibodies against gluten cross over the placenta to the baby. This puts the infant at risk of developing a leaky gut, inflammation and food sensitivities even before its birth. It's not difficult to explain the surge in the number of congenital thyroid disorders, Type 1 diabetes, autism, attention-deficit disorder and attention-deficit hyperactive disorder, to name a few.

A recent study in Belgium found that black carbon particles collected in the lungs of pregnant women and crossed over through the placenta, accumulating on the side facing the growing foetus.[10] In another study, co-published by Dr Noel Mueller in Boston in 2018, the children of women exposed to higher levels of particulate matter in their third trimester were significantly more likely to have high blood pressure. This was mediated through inflammation, secondary to a leaky gut.

During the prenatal period, there are unique inflammatory changes in maternal gut function. If the gut becomes leaky, it can even result in pregnancy loss—because the permeability allows immune triggers to leak into the bloodstream. Maternal malnutrition can not only alter gut permeability of the baby but also affect development and alter gene expression. This can have long-term implications for the offspring. Maternal obesity also negatively impacts the offspring in the same way.[11]

22. **Pregnancy, Breastfeeding and Post-Pregnancy**: The times when the woman's body undergoes hormonal changes (like pregnancy and post-pregnancy, menstruation and menopause) have an impact on her gut. This could be because of the effect of hormones on gut flora, causing an increased permeability. It's therefore not surprising that during the postnatal period, women find it difficult to lose weight and develop thyroid disorders, joint pains, mood swings and even post-partum depression. An understanding of the importance of gut function is why traditional practices of mother care after childbirth focus heavily on digestion and special diets.

Breastfeeding too imparts a huge early advantage to developing a healthy microbiome compared to formula feed. A special species called bifidobacterium gets in through breast milk, which is one of the critical types of bacteria for a healthy gut and immune system.

23. **Perimenopause and Postmenopause**: Menopause doesn't only affect women's reproductive abilities, create mood swings and cause weight

gain, it also negatively impacts their gut health. During the perimenopause phase, the body produces less oestrogen, which helps regulate the stress hormone cortisol. Increased cortisol slows down digestion and can create an imbalance in gut flora.

A collection of gut microbes called the oestrobolome modulates the circulation of oestrogens, thus affecting their levels. In a healthy gut, the oestrobolome produces the requisite amounts to maintain oestrogen balance. In an unbalanced gut microbiome, these levels get disturbed and induce a leaky gut, as do age-related oestrogen imbalances. Inflammatory disorders kick in during these phases because of these changes.

24. **Places and Time Zones**: Different places and populations have different gut microbiomes. When we relocate, eat local food and drink water and other beverages, our gut flora gets impacted by the change. It's hardly surprising that people say their bowel functions change when they visit other places. Some of these changes can affect the gut flora balance and cause permeability.

Travel too is hard on our digestive systems and gut. Long flights are dehydrating, the food often contains preservatives, and the time zone difference means that we eat at times that are not in sync with our diurnal rhythms. Recent studies have shown that melatonin also interacts with the immune system and has positive immunological effects, mediated through an altered gut microbiome.

Lifestyle Factors

25. **Pressure, Problems and Stress:** The gut–brain connection is a fact; it's called the Gut–Brain Axis. When we 'feel' emotions, good or stressful, we feel them first in the gut (as explained in Chapter I). And the connection works the other way too; when the gut is disturbed, it can send signals to the brain and create stress. So, stress leads to a distressed gut and vice versa.

    Even short-term exposure to stress can impact the microbiota by altering the proportion of flora varieties and, in turn, changes in the gut microbiome influence stress response, anxiety and depression. Within the past decade, it has become clear that the gut microbiota is a key regulator of the gut–brain axis.

26. *Pranayama* **and Low Oxygen:** Pranayama helps increase inner calm, both mentally and in the gut. Yogic breathing techniques of pranayama help the gut–brain connection to work better by stimulating the vagus nerve, the longest cranial nerve, which runs from the brain stem to the abdomen.

    Low oxygen levels (also called hypoxia) are pro-inflammatory: according to Dr Warburg, when there is anaerobic respiration (without oxygen), metabolic efficiency falls and detoxification is poor (this is called the Warburg Effect); it creates inflammation, adversely impacts gut flora, and predisposes the individual to a leaky gut. It's a precursor to disorder and disease.

27. **Passive Entertainment, Technology:** Everything today seems to be available at the touch of a button, or a screen. Work was already desk-bound for most people, for many hours in the day, and now, shopping, education and certainly entertainment has moved from being a moderate physical activity to a front-of-screen one (this has been exacerbated with the onset of COVID-19). Many of these habits are formed in childhood, so inactivity among children is worrying.

When we stare at screens at work and come home and become couch potatoes, and spend our evenings lolling on a La-Z-Boy, we are not doing our gut any favours. Sedentary time, which refers to the amount of time one is inactive, has been linked to the development of a distinct path towards ill health, impacted gut flora, and can trigger the development of a leaky gut. As a matter of fact, sitting is also called the 'New Tobacco'; **each** extra hour of TV-watching per day increases inflammatory-related deaths by 11 per cent and the risk of dying from cardiovascular disease by 18 per cent, according to a Melbourne study published in the *Journal of the American Heart Association* in 2012. 'The human body was designed to move, not sit for extended periods of time,' said the study's lead author, Professor David Dunstan from the Baker Heart and Diabetes Institute. The researchers monitored the viewing habits of 8800 adults over six years before publishing the results.

The answer: Move more and move more often!

28. **Physical Activity, Too Much or Too Little:** Lack of exercise impacts our gut adversely—both overtly and covertly. On the visible angle, we gain weight; more worryingly, it can be around the abdomen. This makes the gut flora go out of sync. Exercise helps increase diversity in beneficial gut bacteria. It also helps in the production of short-chain fatty acids that are linked to a healthier gut and longevity. A systemic review of ten studies reported a higher prevalence of beneficial bacteria active among inactive individuals, especially athletes.[12]

But you can have too much of a good thing. According to a meta-review of twenty previous studies on exercise and gut health by a team from Monash University and the University of Tasmania, overexercising can trigger cells in the gut into leaking toxins into the bloodstream.

29. **Parties, Alcohol, Excesses and Eating Out:** Eating out, eating calorie-rich food, eating late and drinking copious amounts of alcohol are very trying on the gut. The problem with parties is the lavish hospitality expected by our culture virtually ensures both dietary excess and late eating. Neither of these is kind to the gut flora.

Heavy alcohol consumption encourages the overgrowth of harmful bacteria and reduces helpful bacteria; this imbalance can cause a leaky gut. On the other hand, studies have found that people who drank red wine had an increased diversity of gut microbiota and favoured good gut flora, implying a protective role. More research is required to fully understand the effect of polyphenols in wine. And remember, excess consumption can surely be counterproductive.

Genetics

30. **Pre-Programmed DNA and Ethnicity (in other Words, Our Genome):** We all have some degree of leaky gut, as the gut barrier is not completely impenetrable. Some of us may have a genetic predisposition and may be more sensitive to changes in the digestive system but our DNA is not the only one to blame, since environmental triggers also interact with the genes. However, ethnic background as well as individual genetic make-up do determine the diversity of gut flora and a predisposition to developing food sensitivities and disorders. The microbiome is, as mentioned earlier, an individual's signature.

The role of genetics and epigenetics in our well-being has evolved to the point that specific genes and their functions have been identified. One important metabolic pathway in the body that is critical to maintaining health is the methylation cycle, which is activated by enzymes.

Glitches and defects in the methylation cycle can lead to (among several other dysfunctions) digestive issues, gastric reflux, food sensitivities and leaky gut.

It's comparable to a domino effect: if one enzyme in the cycle doesn't line up properly, it affects the next one in the queue and the next. From low folate levels to high histamines and repair of the gut lining—these are all functions that can contribute to developing other sensitivities, detoxification defects, inflammation, cancer and immune dysregulation.

Others

31. **Parasites, Post-Surgery, Illness and Trauma:** We can't avoid surgery or illness, but it's important to know that post-surgery trauma can lead to a change in gut flora, which is worsened by drugs and antibiotics. Also, gut flora balance can determine the risk of developing infections such as candida and parasites, which in turn can affect the permeability of our gut. In fact, the gut microbiome of critically injured patients undergoes significant changes in the first seventy-two hours after injury. Signs of candidiasis include redness and itching in moist areas of the body, such as the vagina, anus and testicles, and also thick toenails, brain fog, mood issues, sinusitis and fatigue.

32. **Parity, Kind of Birth:** The term *para* refers to births. *Primipara* is a woman who has given birth for the first time and *multipara*, more than one time. Every time a woman goes through hormonal changes, it affects the gut. The more the number of such upheavals, the greater the chances of developing a leaky gut. This can be worsened by the use of hormones, antibiotics and drugs during pregnancy.

The kind of birth also matters. Naturally-born babies get the benefit of the flora in the vagina; those born via C-Section do not. In mammals, colonization of the infant's gut is thought to largely begin at birth, when delivery through the birth canal exposes the infant to its mother's vaginal microbiome, thereby initiating a critical maternal influence over the baby's lifelong flora.[13] Research shows that microbiota influences almost every aspect of a person's health throughout life.

In fact, C-section infants are now wrapped with the mother's vaginal swabs just to make up for this lack. C-Sections are also hard on the mother because of the use of antibiotics, etc. This makes her gut flora go out of sync, the impact of which can be passed to the infant through breast milk. This puts them at a higher risk of developing chronic health problems, including metabolic disorders, obesity, autoimmunity allergies and mental health issues.

33. **Protective Vaccines:** There is no denying that vaccinations are important to protect us against many diseases. This is also a two-way relationship: the gut microbiome affects vaccination response and vaccinations can affect the gut microbiome. An illustrative case is that of a twenty-two-year-old man who developed multiple sclerosis after something as innocuous as a tetanus shot. Anecdotal evidence has linked the development of autism to a neurodevelopmental disorder soon after the administration of the MMR vaccine shot. Although robust data does not support this association, the link cannot be ignored and a protective gut-healing diet must be initiated pre and post vaccination. This is especially important for those who are at a higher risk or have a positive family history of autoimmune disorders.

34. **Piecemeal Rather than Holistic Approach:** When you fall ill, you end up going to a gastroenterologist, a cardiologist, a neurologist, a dermatologist, etc. This piecemeal approach to sickness and health means that, depending on your symptoms, your actual disorder is a mix of several issues; they are all part of the same body. **And they are all connected to your gut.**

   This patchy treatment rather than a holistic approach has led to patients consuming more drugs, leading to leaky gut and food sensitivities. A patient goes through several specialists, tests and medications, and often, the primary reasons for ill health get missed. A general practitioner or functional medicine expert can work better to join the dots and understand the real problem. Together with the medicines, their side effects, the tests and anxiety can lead to changes in gut flora, developing leaky gut and inflammation. This usually worsens the problem rather than resolving it.

35. **Peace and Prayer**: While stress alters the microbiome, which leads to a leaky gut and increased levels of colonic inflammation, meditation and prayer are gaining popularity in clinical settings to help reduce stress. Research supports the fact that they help regulate stress response, thereby suppressing chronic inflammation and maintaining a healthy gut barrier function. Scientists today recommend the integration of meditation into wellness models.

    Prayer and meditation activate the pineal gland (a small, pea-sized gland in the middle brain), which releases anti-inflammatory hormones like melatonin. This controls our circadian rhythms and reproductive hormones. According to Vedic thought and other traditional philosophies in ancient cultures, the pineal gland opens 'the third eye', leading to the enhancement of intuition and telepathy. Keeping the gut–brain axis in mind, the impact of meditation in maintaining good gut health is obvious. While one cannot do without modern technologies, when their use is too aggressive, it may tilt the balance and adversely impact health.

Geopathic stress refers to the relationship between the Earth's energies and people's well-being. Among others, it includes electromagnetic instability, radiation, satellite towers, electrical poles and even smog levels. All of these are new areas of conversation, and so far, scientifically unproven, but may be impacting inflammation and gut flora.

Whether or not they do, and in what quantity, is not known. What is known, however, is that meditation and prayer help the mind achieve inner peace. And peace of mind is often the most important part of peace in the gut.

PART II

What Should We Do?

*'Those who think they have no time for healthy eating
will sooner or later have to find time for illness'*
—Edward Stanley, Lord Derby

Our mental and intellectual development is directly
related to the quality of our food intake.

Chapter VIII

Food for Thought

'Yatha Annam, Tatha Manam'
—Ancient Indian scriptural maxim

'If music be the food of love, play on,' says the lovesick Duke Orsino in Shakespeare's *Twelfth Night*. To turn around the phrase, however, might be more apt; very often, for most of us, 'Food Is the Music of Love.'

Indeed, a love of food exists in all of us. And why not? We eat not just for pleasing our taste buds, but also for other senses, such as sight and smell. We also eat with our hearts, for emotional reasons. The irritability when we are starving, hungry and angry, has a term—it's called Hangry. We eat when we are happy, when we are sad, tired, lonely, and we love to eat with others. As George Bernard Shaw said, 'There is no love sincerer than the love of food', a comment I think resonates with all of us.

Food = Mood

Awareness of the close bond between food and mood was well-known to the ancients. From Ayurveda to Chinese medicine, practitioners have always been aware that what we eat affects us both physically and emotionally. Ayurveda, an over-5000-year-old science, promotes well-being through the belief that nutrition is not just for the body but also nourishment for the mind and the soul. In ancient Chinese medicine, food is divided into natures and an excess of any kind creates an imbalance in the body and the mind. I think that though the relationship between food and mood is an extremely close one, it's also quite a fragile one; it's very easy to tilt the balance in the wrong direction when we let cravings get the better of us.

Our Brain: No Off Switch

The brain, like the heart, never sleeps. So, it needs constant fuel to function—but to function well, it requires quality nutrition. Research over the last two decades has brought a deepened understanding of brain chemistry, together with the effect of food on behaviour and mental health. Certain nutrients in food alter the neurochemical messengers called neurotransmitters, which help brain function and carry signals between nerve cells.[1]

The Big Three

The three main neurotransmitters associated with food are dopamine, norepinephrine and serotonin. While dopamine and norepinephrine are associated with alertness, serotonin has a calming, relaxing and feel-good effect. These neurotransmitters are produced in the brain from components of food. Foods that contain vitamins, minerals and antioxidants nourish the brain. **Highly-processed, low-nutrient-value foods, or foods that have high quantities of refined sugar, promote insulin resistance, inflammation and oxidative stress.** This impairs brain function and can set off mood disorders and altered eating behaviour, as has been said in the first half of the book.

Endorphins, another set of feel-good neurotransmitters, positively influence mood and appetite and decrease pain sensitivity and stress. They are produced by the brain (pituitary gland). The word *endorphin* comes from putting together the words 'endogenous', meaning from within the body, and morphine, an opiate pain reliever. Endorphins are released during starvation (including fasting for many hours) and by prolonged exercise.

Changes in the levels of these neurotransmitters lead to an alteration in mood. Foods high in carbohydrate content increase the production of an amino acid called tryptophan, a precursor of serotonin. It's why people often crave carbohydrate-rich foods like sweets, desserts, bread, rice, roti and pasta and eat them as comfort foods. Interestingly, the spike in serotonin also explains the drowsiness that sets in after eating a carbohydrate-rich meal. In fact, the effect goes beyond calming. Often called the 'happiness' chemical, serotonin helps uplift mood, reduces anxiety and makes us feel happy. It also has a role in regulating appetite by increasing satiety. In the gut, serotonin regulates bowel function and movement.

To give you a food–mood example, take chocolate: we love it and crave it—but that is not just because it's delicious. Chocolate contains tryptophan (an amino acid in chocolate); its consumption increases the release of serotonin and endorphins. The fat and phenylalanine aid endorphin release. It also contains tyrosine, an amino acid that is the precursor to dopamine—a chemical that controls the brain's reward and pleasure centre. No wonder it is a food for comfort, pleasure and love, and was even considered a sacred food by ancient civilizations like the Mayans.

Blood Sugar and Mood

Another way in which food influences mood is its effect on blood sugar levels; a drop in blood sugar (hypoglycemia) can cause irritability, anxiety, fatigue and mood swings. Nutrient and vitamin deficiencies are common in those with abnormal blood glucose levels and these deficiencies can also have an impact on mood. Severe chronic deficiencies of vitamin B6, B12, folic acid, thiamine, niacin, vitamin C and magnesium can cause irritability, mood swings, panic and anxiety attacks. Deficiencies of micronutrients including iron, copper, zinc and antioxidants impair neurotransmitter synthesis. Researchers have found that inadequate levels of magnesium can result in damage to the brain's nerve cells and lead to mood disorders.

Intolerance and Mood Swings

Food sensitivities also trigger mood changes. Evidence is accumulating that food sensitivity (to gluten and dairy) can trigger mood swings, anxiety, fatigue, depression, aggressive behaviour and other disorders. Intolerance to lactose, a sugar in dairy products, can cause irritability, anxiety and aggressiveness in children. Exactly how it does this is still not clear, but probably exorphins are involved. Exorphins are exogenous (not produced by our bodies) opioid peptides produced by proteins like gluten and casein (dairy protein). They are involved in controlling cravings and eating behaviour as well as in producing symptoms of schizophrenia, autism and other psychological disorders like depression, anxiety and mood swings.

Our brains' reward/opioid centres release dopamine, which encourages us to eat more and hence have difficulty in giving it up. And when we are on an elimination diet, even exposure to small amounts creates a relapse into the same eating behaviour pattern as before.

'The Cure Is in the Cause Itself!'

Gut–Brain Connect

As I have shared in Chapter I, the gut is the body's second brain. And the gut and the brain work closely together. For every message sent out by the brain to the gut, there are nine sent by the gut to the brain.[2] The enteric nervous system is often referred to as the second brain or the gut–brain, and it is home to over 100 million neurons woven through the gut lining. Researchers have determined that 95 per cent of serotonin and about 50 per cent of dopamine are produced in the gut—both these neurotransmitters influence mood as well as mobility in the gastrointestinal tract. Gut bacteria produce these and other transmitters but, interestingly, are also influenced by these chemicals, which suggests interdependence.

Researchers believe that gut bacteria communicate with the brain via the vagus nerve. In cases where this nerve is severed, bacterial influence on the brain is not active. Studies in mice[3] show that disease-causing bacteria can alter their brain chemistry, making them bolder or more anxious and afraid. This reveals the strong connection between dysbiosis and mood. When mice were given probiotics such as lactobacillus, the levels of corticosterone and depression reduced when they were placed in stressful situations.

In fact, diets for neurodevelopmental disorders like autism have centred on the elimination of gluten (wheat protein) and casein (dairy protein) because of the connection between gut flora imbalance and neuro disorders.[4] However, this must not be initiated without the supervision of a qualified physician.

What Do Cravings Signal?

It's normal to crave something once in a while when one is tired, stressed or depressed, but when the craving is compelling and regular, it may signal a nutritional deficiency, an imbalance in your diet, such as too much sugar or carbohydrates, or gut-related issues. Or most likely, a combination of all three.

Nutrition chemistry also teaches us that cheat food helps you climb out of the mood hollows, but the effect **doesn't last**. In the long term, one cannot use—and abuse—food to keep the blues at bay. Food rich in sugars gives a temporary high, but, like any drug, the high is followed by a low—which needs more of the same food. It's diminishing marginal returns in the worst possible way.

When we clean up our diets and remove the offending substances, the first effect is an increase in anxiety as the withdrawal symptoms kick in. Food addictions are like any other addictions; while not overtly dangerous, they definitely push us into ill health.

FACT: *You don't need to **Wrestle** with your **Willpower!*** When you give up sugar, you initially feel edgy, as your threshold of sweetness changes. But then, even unsweetened milk seems sweet—you can train your palate.

You need the awareness that eating healthy food **can** and **does** spike happiness levels. A diet consistent with the right food choices creates long-term improvement in physical and mental health. The Mediterranean diet is famous for stabilizing mood because of its fruit- and vegetable-rich content and omega-3 fats. In fact, after altering eating habits, many clients come back and report feeling encouraging changes in their emotions:

'*Bada achha* feel *kar rahe hain* [We are feeling very good]', and '*Hamara* mood *bada* positive *hai*' [Our mood is very positive]. They are simply observing their own change in mood, but the science behind this backs it up.

FACT: *You Really Are What You Eat!* This isn't just a saying; it's quite a profound statement of fact. As Jean Savarin, a French lawyer and epicure, famously said, 'Tell me what you eat and I'll tell you who you are.' If you understand the depth of the connection between food, mood and health, you can establish a healthy relationship with food.

Break the bad mood cycle and stay in the good mood food zone.

Chapter IX

Action Plan: Composing a Chef d'Oeuvre

'If the doctor of today does not become the dietician of tomorrow, the dietician of today will become the doctor of tomorrow'
—Dr Alexis Carrel, Rockefeller Institute of Medical Research

Music begins with folk; when the notes get organized into specific rules or disciplines, they become a raga. Just like music, our world is replete with food items; they are the notes in the 'music of food'. Nutrition science is the instrument that strings the notes to arrive at the composition of dietary ragas.

And sensible rules of eating are deeply entrenched in our culture, over centuries of experience from our forefathers. When we apply these rules carefully to food and how it is eaten, it becomes a diet. When we ignore them in our desire to constantly tickle the palate, there is dietary chaos.

This is the very foundation of composing a diet. We need to combine the food notes correctly. Strung together in a manner that's pleasant in its effect on the body, they result in a melodious harmony and nourish the body and soul, just like a perfectly composed raga. Poor food choices and habits are like badly-strung notes, they create a discordant cacophony in the body's functions.

And, just as there are different ragas for different times and moods, diets differ for body types. There is **NO** one-size-fits-all diet plan. Another aspect of diet is that we think the word 'diet' has a shelf life—that we can go on one, reach a goal and then resume old eating patterns. The fact is that the word comes from the Greek *diaita,* which translates to 'a way of life'.

The first important step is **AST: Assessment, Testing** and **Starting** your journey.

1. **Assessment:** When and how does one know if one has a leaky gut or food sensitivity? The **red flags** include:
    *   You have obvious signs and symptoms, like frequent allergies or abdominal bloating.
    *   You've tried but haven't been able to reach your health goals. More often than not, common concerns are around:
        *   **Body weight or shape:** it could be the inability to achieve adequate weight loss or reduce belly fat even with frugal eating

and regular exercise. Or being unable to gain weight. For some, it's not being able to build muscle mass despite working out.

- **Metabolic syndrome:** high cholesterol, diabetes, high blood pressure and high uric acid.
- **Health concerns:** common complaints include digestive disorders, poor energy, fatigue, sleep disorders, mood issues, anxiety and depression. Common digestive disorders include IBS, hyperacidity, reflux, constipation, diarrhoea and vomiting.
- **Skin and hair issues:** hair fall, dull skin and rashes, acne and dandruff, despite a good diet and supplements.
- **Either personal or family history** of autoimmune disorders such as thyroid disorders, multiple sclerosis, joint pain, arthritis, lupus, polymyositis (a degeneration of the muscles), liver disease and kidney disorders.
- **Neurological complaints** such as neuropathy, numbness and tingling in extremities and epilepsy.
- History of **anaemia, osteoporosis** and **nutritional deficiencies**.
- History or family history of **cancer** tumours.
- History of **psychological** or **psychiatric issues**: depression, anxiety, schizophrenia, mood swings, ADD, ADHD, brain fog.

♦ **Gestational diabetes, PCOS, difficulties in conception or history of miscarriages**.

♦ **Nagging complaints** that do not respond to treatment: frequent colds, fevers, sinus and other infections, easy fractures and injuries, asthma or other respiratory issues.

2. **Testing**: Often, to truly discover what works for us, we need to first learn what works against us. To identify these triggers, we need professional help. Don't be afraid to seek such help. Through serology (blood tests) and the planned elimination of a number of foods and then reintroduction of items one by one, our personal food nemeses can be identified. As explained in Part I of this book, the effect of any one or all of the four Gs can cause an imbalance in the gut microbiome and a leaky gut. If you have any of the issues mentioned above in the assessment process, that merits a deep dive to look inside your gut for food sensitivities. The method is:

• **Simple blood tests** under the supervision of a qualified professional. They can help establish your food sensitivities or deficiencies.

• **Testing for Wheat Sensitivity**: this is usually a test for IgA and IgG antibodies. They show evidence of celiac disease or non-celiac wheat sensitivity (NCWS). Currently, available IgG tests include several food items as a panel. These are done as a leaky gut allows many other commonly-eaten foods to cross the intestinal barrier. If the body makes antibodies against them, they may also be contributing to the symptoms even if they haven't been the original trigger food.

With this information, your customized diet plan can be drawn up. The primary culprits include wheat gluten-containing grains such as barley and rye, as well as cross-reacting grains (corn, soya, oats, buckwheat and amaranth). But, before drawing up any restrictive or long-term, gluten-free diet, the tests should be carried out to see if there is NCWS or celiac disease.

3. **Starting** your food journey: Setting out on this voyage within takes time, patience and discipline. There will be new learnings—but ones with rich dividends.

    Any dive into the functioning of your gut begins with analysis: you remove certain foods and then reintroduce them, one by one. Maintain a food and symptom diary. Reactions can start immediately or take up to seven days. Usually, symptoms tend to peak around Day Two. Antibodies can stay positive for up to three months: anything beyond 20 ppm (parts per million) is recognized by our immune system. Since none of us can remember everything we eat beyond a day or two, the only way to keep track of the association between consumption and reaction is to keep a food diary. Remember that even small amounts of eliminated foods contamination can lead to symptoms.

    Every stage in this journey is a step towards **Healing the Leaky Gut.**

The process of **healing** is summarized in a **4 R Protocol**. It's a systematic and comprehensive method that not only improves the systems of the body but also heals them—to achieve long-term well-being. This method has helped thousands of my clients achieve their health and fitness goals.

Healing the leaky gut can resolve minor and major digestive disorders like the ones mentioned earlier in this chapter (hyperacidity, acid reflux, constipation, diarrhoea, vomiting, constipation and bloating) as well as ulcerative colitis, Crohn's disease and IBS. It can also help alleviate symptoms related to gut health, such as acne, anxiety, autoimmune conditions, brain fog, fatigue, joint and muscle pain, chronic headaches, migraines and more. Since the digestive tract is where most of the immune cells are and where one absorbs nutrients, improving gut health derives health benefits across body functions. It's not surprising that many of my patients have not only managed their diabetes but also reversed it. Other medical conditions, from hypertension to metabolic syndrome, neuropathies, nephropathies, infertility and PCOS, have all been treated. (Chapter XIII details illustrative case studies on a list of conditions.) However, please note, these results are obtained only under the supervision of a qualified professional.

The steps in the 4 R Protocol are:

R1: Remove (sensitive foods and elements)
R2: Replace (with appropriate alternatives)

R3: Rebuild (nutrients and the gut lining)
R4: Restore (gut function and rebalance gut microbiota)

R1. Step One is the elimination or **Removal** of foods that activate your immune system to produce antibodies and cause inflammation. Research shows that the most common foods that trigger antibody reactions contain gluten; they must be religiously removed from your diet. So, in the first phase, you need to eliminate wheat in all its forms and gluten-containing grains like barley, rye and spelt, and also follow the grain science (remove grains like corn, oats, soya and buckwheat). The reason is, many people who react adversely to gluten have a cross-reaction to these cereals as well, and they should be removed in the first stage. Cross-reactivity occurs when the proteins found in the foods are similar, so the immune system sees them as the same and reacts similarly to them.

- There is also a need to remove any other foods that can irritate the gut: reducing or eliminating alcohol, coffee, processed food and food additives is advisable.
- People with a leaky gut may also have issues with carbohydrates in milk (lactose) or sugars in fruit.
- They may have developed sensitivity or allergies to certain foods such as nuts.
- Once the diet is started, the positive effects kick in; medication may need to be reviewed by your doctor.

- Infections via bacteria, parasites and other pathogens need to be looked at.

R2. Replace: Just removing inflammatory grains, however, is not enough—the next step is to **Replace** them with appropriate healthy alternatives that are kinder on the gut. These may include any of the following—rice, millets, quinoa, teff, lentil or nut flours (e.g., almond, coconut, etc.). Millets are coarse grain and make good alternative flours if blended with low glycaemic flours. While white rice is the most common, unpolished brown, red and black rice are also becoming popular. These forms of rice have the nutritional advantage of having higher fibre content (a prebiotic benefit) than polished white rice and they have more nutrients. However, some of the permitted grains can cause irritation in some of those who have a more severe condition or can be contaminated with wheat by virtue of a common flour mill.

Rice and some other foods do have a high glycaemic index (GI), so can be counterproductive in terms of inflammation. Their use needs to be balanced out with the addition of other, low glycaemic flours. Millets include ragi, bajra, jowar, sama and rajgira, among others. Teff is a seed grass native to Africa and quinoa is a seed native to South America that have gained traction as alternative cereals. Pulse or lentil flours are besan, moong dal, etc. A diet that contains rice, pulse and millet flours helps improve the glycaemic index and thus the insulin response. This is also the best way to raise the quality of protein. Grain science by itself will not work unless the replacements are healthy and the overall diet is well-chosen.

R3. Rebuild and Repair the gut. This requires replenishing it with micronutrients and gut-healing herbs. Some of you who suffer from chronic digestive issues have an insufficiency of certain elements that are key to digestion, such as stomach acid and digestive enzymes. You may also be deficient in nutrients. Your gut-healing plan may include:

- Enzyme supplements to replace the missing elements that help better digestion of fats, carbohydrates and proteins.
- Foods containing components that help the body produce these enzymes: examples are bitter foods or raw papaya, which is an excellent source of enzyme-rich food.
- Foods and/or supplements to address nutrient deficiencies.

The role of enzymes in repairing and rebuilding the gut must be emphasized. They are protein-like substances that act as catalysts in the chemical reactions that power body function: digestion, pumping of the heart, breathing and more. The body produces digestive enzymes, but with age and stress, this production can get compromised. Inadequate enzyme function can lead to poor gut function—and this impacts overall body health.

There are three categories of enzymes that are involved in the digestive process—for the three main nutrient categories:

- Amylases, which help digest carbohydrates into simple sugars,
- Proteases, which break down proteins into amino acids, and
- Lipases, which digest fats into fatty acids.

Our bodies produce the enzymes they need (some are produced by the pancreas, the stomach, the saliva and even the intestines), but there are factors that reduce their production. These include overuse of drugs, excess alcohol, stress, smoking, toxic substances in the environment such as pesticides and polluted air and water, and even age itself.

For those who have digestive disorders, an enzyme-rich diet helps manage them better by optimizing gut functionality. This can be achieved by adding foods rich in natural digestive enzymes (raw, fermented or very lightly cooked foods) or supplementing them with the addition of probiotics. Enzyme supplementation therapy is an important tool in treating many digestive disorders as well as malabsorption.

Digestive enzymes are destroyed by heat, so overcooking or processing reduces their content. In fact, modern urban diets are high in processed foods, industrially-manufactured bakery and snack products, frozen foods, dehydrated foods and overcooked vegetables. All of these are low in enzyme content. We need to include enzyme-rich natural and supplemented foods to improve overall gut health.

In this repair phase, the idea is to create an environment that supports gut healing and long-term relief. Another activity that helps rebuild gut flora balance is fasting, which will be detailed in the next chapter. We facilitate the repair of the intestinal cells and mucosa, lower inflammation and help the microbiome find a happy home within our digestive tract. We may include foods high in vitamins A, C, D and E as well as the mineral zinc; foods rich in amino acids, such as desi ghee or bone broth; foods and supplements such as rice congee, honey, aloe vera, curcumin, apple puree, bone broth, marshmallow, slippery elm, psyllium husk, L-glutamine (an amino acid supplement that helps in repairing a leaky gut) and collagen (a protein that helps repair the damaged gut). The body manufactures both L-glutamine and collagen, but supplements of these products are useful in times of stress.

The rest of your lifestyle must be changed according to the **thirty-five Ps** laid out in Chapter VII, to avoid triggers that injure the gut and to support the healing process.

R4. Restore: Once symptoms have improved significantly, the final phase is to **Restore** the balance in the gut microbiome (the collection of good gut bacteria that play a leading role in maintaining immune, digestive and metabolic health). It's important to keep these bugs happy by adding:

- **Prebiotic foods:** Prebiotics are the type of food that gut bacteria love and they help them grow and multiply. They include psyllium husk (isabgol), onions, garlic, leeks, asparagus, apples and bananas, to name some. They produce butyric acid in the gut (by promoting the growth of bacteria that generate it). Butyric acid is the short-chain fatty acid that is the predominant fuel for the gut cells—high-fibre foods encourage its production in the gut.
- **Probiotic foods:** Probiotic foods are rich in microorganisms that are beneficial for our digestive system—but they must reach the gut alive and in a certain concentration. Fermented foods such as yogurt, apple cider vinegar, pickled vegetables, kanji, honey, sauerkraut, kimchi and kombucha (make sure you check that the grains/starter used conforms to the grain and dairy science) are excellent. Adequate hydration is critical to deriving the benefits of the above.

The restoration and rebalance of gut flora is a process that addresses the harmony of function in all the body's systems. In order to effectively reset the elements of health—physical, mental, social and spiritual—we need to be aware of the enormous influence our lifestyle and habits have on the gut and the body.

Healthy eating is not a limited-time affair, but a consistent habit.

Chapter X

No Shortcuts: The Directive Principles of Dietary Policy

Self-Sabotage Is the Worst Sabotage—How to Stick To Your Diet and Not Fall off the Wagon

Just as the Indian Constitution lays out the Directive Principles of State Policy, the values and codes that provide direction to the body politic, there are some fundamental principles that should govern the human body's dietary programme too. If you follow these directives of dietary policy carefully, they provide a blueprint that will guide you towards health and well-being.

Part I of this book has detailed the relevant scientific information that you need to know. To quickly recap, Part I includes:

1. It's not your fault. The ecosystem outside changed our insides.
2. The realization that consistent poor eating habits are making people unhealthy, unhappy or simply out of shape!
3. The awareness that optimum gut function is integral to maintaining healthy functions in your body.
4. The understanding that, when gluten and glucose in your diet combine with actions in the gut and create intestinal permeability (a leaky gut), this creates central obesity or girth—this is the **4 G** effect that is responsible for inflammation, ill health, disorder and disease.
5. The knowledge that your very own, personal *brahmastra* to heal the gut and begin the journey to better health is **what, when and how you choose to eat.**

Centenarian Secrets

> '*Oh Lord, let me die young, as late as possible*'
> —A Greek prayer

Before we get to the principles underpinning dietary policy, let's take a look at the longest-lived communities in the world: the centenarians of Okinawa in Japan, the Hunza people of North-west Pakistan, the Sardinians and Ikarias of the Mediterranean, the Vilcabambans of South America and the Abkhazians of the Caucasus.

Ikaria in Greece is called the island of long life, the Hunza valley in north Pakistan has been considered the original Shangri La, and the longevity of residents of Vilcabamba in Ecuador and of Abkhazia in southern Russia is legendary. Incidence of diseases such as high blood pressure, cardiovascular disease and diabetes are virtually nil, as are cases of arthritis, Alzheimer's or cancer.

These are also called the 'Blue Zones', named for the blue circles researchers drew on the map to delineate some of the oldest and healthiest communities in the world.

How is this possible? These communities are separated by oceans and climate and have many social differences.

Divided by continents and cultures, these varied populations are, however, united by similarities in their **diet and lifestyle**. Not the actual dishes—they are in vastly different areas of the world. But their longevity is strongly linked with the kind of food choices they make, the clean environments they live in and the amount and kind of exercise they are used to: low-calorie, healthy diets, plus plenty of outdoor physical activity and access to clean air.

As a matter of fact, nations where traditional patterns of eating are still intact, like Japan, are home to high numbers of centenarians even today. Caloric restriction is a hallmark of longevity because it can modulate genes linked to a longer life span.

Simple Unities

The common thread in their diet is that it is rich in fruits and vegetables, fish or plant protein, whole grains, healthy fats and good water; low in meats, refined grain flours and sugars; and does not contain toxic industrial trans fats. They do not consume chemical-laden, processed or pesticide-loaded food. Familial closeness and physically-active lifestyles are also features of these long-lived people.

What the experience of these centenarians tells us is that there are absolutely **no shortcuts and no alternatives** to formulating a healthy eating plan. But it is also a pointer to the fact that, provided you ring in real dietary change, at any age, it can help reverse some—if not all—of the effects of earlier poor food choices. In other words, 'It's Never Too Late!'

Is achieving the centenarians' lifestyle difficult? Quite the contrary. **Actually, it's the very simplicity of it that is the greatest gift they have to give us.** You do not need massive doses of supplements and extensive medication to accomplish good health goals; neither do you need expensive and complicated therapy to live long and to live healthy.

The key is already with us. Apply the **KIS** principle: Keep It Simple!

Did I hear 'It's easier said than done?' Not true!

CLUB MED: SUPERIOR DIET?

The term 'Mediterranean diet' implies a singular cuisine, but it's a misnomer. It includes Italian, French, Greek and Spanish cuisines, among others. But they do have commonalities: they are based on olive oil, plenty of fruits and vegetables, dairy, wine and omega-3-rich fatty fish. They are relatively low in carbohydrates and rich in antioxidants and fibre. The region is also conservative in the use of pesticides and genetically-modified seeds. There is an emphasis on locally-grown food. Air and water pollution are less. All these have a profound impact on food quality.

The Paradox: The Mediterranean diet is rich in animal fats and cholesterol, yet the incidence of heart disease is low. The reason is that in diets, the quality of the fats matters more than the quantity. Omega-3 fats from fish, walnuts and leafy vegetables are anti-inflammatory.

How can Indians achieve a Mediterranean-like diet? By switching to omega-3-rich mustard and sesame oils and adding natural fats from nuts, seeds, desi ghee, butter and coconut oil. We should also avoid foods high in hydrogenated fats (bakery products, namkeens). Cereals should be from mixed grains and pulses to improve insulin response. And there should be fruits and vegetables, preferably locally grown.

Understanding Food Groups

One cardinal principle that must be applied is an understanding of food groups. For ease of communication in this book, I will refer to them just a little differently from the conventional formats. The reason is that any typical plate of food has items that straddle more than one clear category. My three main groups can be categorized as Proteins, Protective Foods and Cereal/Carbohydrates.

Proteins: The building blocks of the body, these can be in the form of plant protein or animal protein, or both. Pulses and legumes are sources of plant protein, and nuts are a source of fats and plant proteins. Meat, fish, poultry, eggs and dairy are all animal proteins.

Protective Foods: This is a rather wide category and includes fruits and vegetables, nuts and seeds, herbs and spices, as well as good fats, fibre and fermented foods and fluids. All of them are protective because they are rich in the vitamins, minerals, antioxidants and fibre that are necessary to achieve health and boost immunity.

Carbohydrates: In this category, grains and cereals form the epicentre from which dietary choices radiate, and are defined by regional preferences (chapatis and other rotis for north India, Pakistan and the Middle East, rice for south India and South-east Asia, pasta for the countries of the Mediterranean, bread for Europe and the US, and so on). They are all carbohydrates, colloquially referred to as 'carbs'. Sugar, sweets and desserts should also be included in this group. From the vegetable pantry, potatoes, sweet potatoes, tapioca and cassava are starchy vegetables that belong best in the carbohydrate category.

In the carbohydrate category, I want to address cereals first. This is because customarily, grains are the staple food that is eaten regularly and in quantity; they tend to dominate the plate in terms of portion size. Carbohydrates fuel the body, giving its cells the energy to perform its work. And once upon a time, most people did a lot of daily physical work and needed the large amount of carbohydrates they consumed (this is true for those who do physical labour even today).

But for most urban Indians, as lifestyles and work patterns have become more sedentary and office-based, the daily carbohydrate requirement has dropped dramatically. Therefore, your diet planning needs to be adjusted for this change in lifestyle, with careful pruning of the daily quantity of cereals and other carbohydrates.

Just adjusting quantity is not enough; you could also be consuming the wrong kind of grains. They could be crops that are farmed with greater reliance on fertilizers and pesticides or highly refined grains. These processes lower the nutritional value of grains and add to the toxic load. If properly planned, a diet low in grain content or even grain-free can be nutritionally sufficient (you need professional help to guide you), provided high-nutrient foods are used as alternatives.

'Gehu khao to phulo [If you eat wheat, you bloat]
Jowar khao to jhoolo [If you eat jowar, you float]'
                                        —Old Gujarati saying

Also, cereals and grains are not the only carbohydrates we consume; whether it's white or brown sugar, jaggery, honey or maple syrup, sugars provide you with extra calories—and no added nutrition (see Chapter V on glucose). It makes sense to very carefully limit our ingestion of sugars. If you have a sweet tooth, then healthy sugars like jaggery, dry fruits and honey are certainly better than refined sugar.

So, attentive planning of the quality, quantity, choice and variety of carbohydrates that are ingested is an important part of the directive principles of healthy eating.

Your choice and quantity of cereal/grain should depend on several relevant factors, which are detailed in the box below.

A GRAIN OF SENSE

The Grain Guide depends on:

- **What Your Gut Can Tolerate:** If you are gluten-sensitive, you can easily replace gluten-containing grains like wheat, barley and rye with others, such as millet flours, sorghum (bajra), quinoa or teff. One warning though: if you need to go gluten-free, it's not enough to simply pick up products that say 'gluten-free'. Many commercially prepared foods may contain too much starch, added sugars or additives.
- **Cross-Reactive Grains:** People who have a gluten sensitivity or intolerance are often also sensitive to grains such as buckwheat (kuttu),

soya, oats, amaranth, spelt or sago (sabudana). This kind of cross-reaction means that ingesting these cereals is likely to create symptoms similar to those caused by gluten. Remember that soya and barley are also not for you. So, if you are gluten-sensitive, carefully remove grains that contain it and see which replacements do not cause the same symptoms. If your gut is too damaged, millets also may be too harsh, initially. Also, about a third of those who cannot tolerate gluten cannot tolerate quinoa too.

- **How Much:** The amount of cereal eaten should depend on your level of physical activity as well as your own weight/waist goals. Also, for those with weight reduction goals, a diet without grains is achievable since you can get your carbohydrate needs fulfilled from sources such as fruits and vegetables, pulses, nuts, seeds and flours of chickpea, almond or other nuts. For most people, one meal should be grain-rich, and one grain-light. The third meal, if eaten at all, should not contain grain and concentrate on protective foods only. However, this may need to be adapted to individual needs.

- **Glycaemic Index (GI):** Wheat and rice are high on the glycaemic index (which ranks carbohydrates according to their effect on blood sugar levels). Low GI flours, such as pulse flours and quinoa, produce a slower increase in blood glucose levels, so they regulate insulin response better—and help control weight.

- **Whole Grains:** Most staples available today are highly refined versions. White rice is highly polished and white wheat flour (maida) is what all bakery products contain. This wasn't always the case: once, wheat was ground whole, along with the nutrient-rich husk, which contained the B vitamins, proteins and natural oils. The refining techniques for wheat, rice and corn have improved their shelf life but removed many nutrients. Whole grains are slower to digest because they have more fibre, which promotes the growth of healthy bacteria in the gut. Whole grains mean getting the whole benefit!

- **Cereal Exchange:** There are many other foods that contain carbohydrates that you may not be factoring into your cereal count. Many snacks (rusks, biscuits, samosas, corn on the cob) are carbohydrate-rich. One serving is one bread roll or a slice of bread, one chapati, half a cup of cooked rice, poha or noodles, two or three biscuits, half a bhatura, one kulcha or one large idli. Two chapatis, one bhatura, one cup of rice or poha are equal to one cereal exchange.

- **Timing:** Timing is critical. When it comes to grain, which one and how much are inextricably linked to what time you consume the grain-rich meal. Your work and lifestyle can help you decide whether that is lunch or dinner—but following the body clock is integral. Cereals should not be consumed after 7 p.m.; only some vegetables or light protein, nuts or fruit.

The other food groups are Proteins and Protective Foods. I am going to talk about them next, along with a third P—Planning; together, these form three significant principles of dietary policy. These three Ps work together as a blueprint that can be used in the journey towards dietary health.

P1: Proteins and Their Pairing: Proteins provide the body with essential body-building elements called amino acids (most of our hormones, neurotransmitters and enzymes are made of these elements). They are so important that you should aim to have two protein-rich meals a day. The protein content in them can be in the form of dals, pulses (or a pancake made from their flour, as in a cheela), soya, nuts or dairy products in case of vegetarians and eggs, meat, chicken or fish for non-vegetarians. **Remember that if you are wheat-sensitive, then soya may not be good for you.**

But it's not enough to merely eat adequate protein; what is very important is to combine these proteins with vegetables. The reason is that proteins leave an acidic residue when digested and vegetables are mostly alkaline. This helps to neutralize the inflammatory and acidic nature of proteins. Vegetables also contain that essential element for the digestive tract—fibre—which proteins lack. The pairing of proteins and vegetables is a match made in digestive heaven!

Sprouts are an excellent source of plant protein; they are low in calories but powerhouses of nutrition. That's because the sprouting process itself increases the levels of nutrients in the seeds. Enzyme-rich, they help the digestive process in the gut and have lower levels of anti-nutrients (compounds that make food difficult to digest). So, it's easier to absorb nutrition from sprouted foods. Sprouted grains are also alkaline, in contrast to the acidic residue left by the grain or pulse in its original form. They are rightly called 'live' or *prana* foods.

There is an ongoing conversation on plant versus animal protein. The simple facts read as follows:

- Both serve equally well, nutritionally.
- Excess consumption of animal protein has a negative effect both on your health and the global ecosystem.
- Animal proteins need more time to digest. They also carry the burden of hormonal and pesticide residue, often more than plant protein.
- If you consume organic, free-range animal protein, do this in moderation.

P2: Protective Foods: Yes, these are vegetables, but also fruit, nuts, tea, seeds, spices and the husks in grains. They are loaded with vitamins, minerals, fibre, phytonutrients and enzymes. Green leafy vegetables and red, yellow and purple ones are packed with phytochemicals and antioxidants. The word 'phyto' may refer to their plant origin, but it truly is a pun— they fight for you!

These protective foods contain plant nutrients and antioxidant compounds like carotenoids and phenolics that are anti-inflammatory and help protect cells from oxidative damage. Devote one meal to the protective plant food group only—it's transformational for the gut.

Value Vegetables: Vegetables are the kings of the diet kingdom; wisdom lies in giving them the biggest share of the plate. Tip: follow the half-plate rule—whenever you fill your plate, ensure that at least half of it is occupied by vegetables. And at least half of the veggies you consume should be either raw, lightly steamed or in soups. Vegetables in their natural or 'live' form contain enzymes, which are destroyed by overcooking.

Vegetables are naturally low in fat and calories—some, like celery, cucumber and radish are calorie-negative, which means they consume more calories being digested than they contain. They are good sources of vitamins and minerals, such as folic acid, vitamins A, B and C, potassium, etc. A veggie-rich diet helps the gut to function well.

Green Power

'Eat your greens' is what mothers have said the world over. Well, they certainly knew their business. Several scientific studies have found that green leafy vegetables provide strong protection against heart disease and chronic degenerative diseases. All brightly-coloured fruits and vegetables contain healthy plant pigments, vitamins and minerals, but greens have the magic one, chlorophyll. It blocks carcinogens by binding to them and making them unavailable to the body. It also helps regenerate critical antioxidants in the body (the production of these decreases with age).

In fact, even red, orange and purple plants are green in the nascent stage and as they ripen, the chlorophyll breaks down and other pigments increase in proportion. When choosing fruits and vegetables, just follow the rainbow. The more brightly-hued your plate, the more phytonutrients you get.

HOW MUCH VEG IS RIGHT?

- Dedicate one meal to just vegetables (or fruit)
- In other meals, half your plate should be full of veggies
- That means five to nine servings a day
- One serving is approx. half a cup
- Total: three to four cups of vegetables every day
- At least half should be raw or lightly cooked

Relish Fruits: Fruits are carbohydrates, yes, but valuable components of the daily diet. They are loaded with vitamins, minerals and phytochemicals that help protect us from disease. The only caveat: since they contain sugar, one to three servings of fruit are adequate.

Dry fruits (raisins, dates, figs, etc.), are excellent fixes for the sweet tooth. Fruit juice should simply be off the table because it contains all the sugar and almost none of the fibre. Packaged fruit juice is anathema to the healthy diet plan; it's packed with extra sugar that can cause an insulin imbalance (which creates inflammation). If you bloat or get gassy after consuming fruit, you may need to look at a low FODMAP diet (refer to FODMAPs in Chapter V).

WHEN TO EAT FRUIT

- Research isn't enough to be conclusive, but traditional food science relies on observed findings.
- Many people who eat fruits after a meal have bloating or flatulence.
- The theory that fruits could ferment while waiting for the gastrointestinal tract to digest everything else that has been eaten with them has merit.
- Best Practice: Eat fruit by itself on an empty stomach or between meals. This is also a concept followed by Ayurveda.

Go Nuts: Nuts (which include walnuts, almonds, pistachios, peanuts, cashews, pine nuts, hazelnuts, macadamia nuts and others) are good sources of fats, proteins and fibre. Most of the fat they contain is anti-inflammatory and heart-healthy. It's a myth that nuts are high-cholesterol foods; they have zero cholesterol. Nut milks and butters can also provide a substitute for those who are intolerant to dairy. Almond and other nut flour can be used instead of wheat as flour in bakery products.

Nuts score high on the satiety index and have a low glycaemic index, so they reduce food cravings and help control blood sugar levels—while providing essential nutrients. They are rich in vitamins and minerals that boost our immune system and are also value food for the brain. Walnuts, for example, look like a mini-brain, don't they?

Seeds too punch well above their weight in goodness. Many seeds are rich in vitamins, minerals, fibre and flavonoids (which fight disease). They also contain the good fats that lower cholesterol (omega-3 fatty acids) and other antioxidants. Sunflower, pumpkin, melon, chia, flax and sesame are some examples of seeds that can provide you with important minerals like magnesium, selenium, copper and zinc. They are small in size, but big in effect; these little powerhouses pack a big immunity-boosting punch.

Spice It Up: You know the saying, 'Variety is the spice of life', right? I think that should be turned around on its head: 'Spice is the variety of life.' Traditionally, Indians—as well as people of other ancient civilizations like the Greeks and the Chinese—have used spices to both improve taste and reduce the inflammatory effect of what we eat. Herbs and spices really should be a few of your favourite things!

The therapeutic value of herbs and spices (see more in Chapter X) comes from their high antioxidant content. Many spices (such as turmeric) are anti-inflammatory. Green chillies, mint, pepper, coriander, cinnamon, cloves, cardamom, thyme, rosemary, basil leaves and basil seeds (sabza), nigella (kalonji) seeds and poppy seeds; these are just a few of the herbs and spices that have health benefits. Black pepper, for instance, was so prized as a condiment that European adventurers vied to find a sea route to India to control the pepper trade!

DAILY DOSE OF GOODNESS

- 2–4 cups of vegetables, raw, steamed or lightly cooked
- 1–2 seasonal fruits
- A variety of nuts
- A handful of herbs
- A fistful of seeds
- A soupçon of spices
- Some sprouts, raw or steamed

Fats: All fats are not equal. There have been many myths about fats, which became perceived wisdom. They have been debunked as more studies have shown that fats are not the true villains of the diet; sugar, as I had mentioned in Part 1 of this book, is a bigger dietary culprit than fats, but has stayed under the radar of the diet police. Some fats are harmful and they should be avoided (see the section headed 'PSST' in Chapter XI). But many fats are not just healthy, they actually improve digestion, gut health and insulin response (see the box below).

HEALTHY FATS: THE GOOD GUYS

Ghee and Butter: Saturated fats have been in the line of fire. But not all saturated fats are equal. Industrially produced saturated fats like margarine and vanaspati are toxic for our bodies. However, this is not true of natural saturated fats like butter and ghee, coconut oil or palm oil. As a matter of fact, our cell membranes are stronger and more stable with saturated fats and cholesterol, which are important for the functionality of the cell.

Ayurvedic detox gives you ghee because it releases toxins from deep within the body and into the gut—for elimination. Grandmas added ghee to our food: on rotis, it reduced their glycaemic index; in times of stress, it gave the gut cells the energy they needed to fight off the release of stress toxins. Butter and ghee contain butyrate, a short-chain fatty acid that also provides the main source of fuel for the cells of the gut lining. To fight off toxins and boost immunity, one needs to provide the soldier cells with energy. Take a good look at our culinary and dietary traditions. Ghee is good for you!

Cold-Pressed Oils: Indigenous cooking mediums like mustard, sesame and coconut oil are excellent sources of good fats. Mustard oil is anti-inflammatory, a source of plant omega-3 and exceptionally good as a flavour enhancer; sesame oil is rich in antioxidants. Olive oil too is loaded with phytonutrients. Remember to use the cold-pressed version of these oils (for other health benefits of coconut oil, see Chapter XII).

Omega-3 fats: These are anti-inflammatory fats. Incidentally, omega-3 fats are not just present in fish (though fatty fish such as salmon are a good source). Vegetarians can enjoy the same benefit by consuming green leafy vegetables, walnuts, flaxseeds, avocados, methi seeds and chia seeds.

HCA: Formatting the Fluids

HCA is an acronym for fluids that are essential for the body to function well—as well as those that we simply enjoy.

Hydrate: The human body is 70 per cent water; adequate hydration, therefore, is essential on a daily basis. Fluids help flush out toxins and are critical to the processes of digestion, elimination and the transport of nutrients. Adequate intake of water and other fluids, such as soups, coconut water, detox water and veggie juice, keeps you from overeating and improves metabolism.

The body cannot dry-clean itself—detox is wet work! But how much fluid do you need? Often, you wait until you're thirsty but, actually, thirst is not the best pointer. By the time you feel thirsty, you may already be somewhat dehydrated. When dehydrated, our brain tires, we feel less alert and more fatigued and it also interferes with sleep patterns.

You need at least 2–2.50 litres of fluid a day, depending on the weather and your activity levels. Also, do not drink excessive water with your meals. It's best to drink a glass or two of water when you wake up, and a glass an hour before and after a meal. Do hydrate during periods of intense exercise. And try to see that the quality of the water you drink is good, preferably alkaline, with good mineral content. If you don't like the taste of plain water, add lemons or ginger or herbs to make it more palatable. Water should be stored in glass or steel bottles, not in plastic ones. Silver, copper and earthen vessels are also excellent ways to store water.

Caffeine: The wake-up drinks of the world, tea and coffee, give us the kick that starts the body's engine. The caffeine in them can be useful for weight loss as they boost energy consumption and efficiency. They also contain polyphenols and minerals. But, like all good things, moderate amounts (two to four cups) are okay. Excess tea and coffee can promote water and mineral loss, as they are diuretics. They also irritate the gut lining because they contain caffeine and tannic acid.

If you love coffee but had to give it a miss because it caused acidity, cold brew coffee offers a way to get the caffeine hit without the heartburn. Cold brew is not hot coffee that has been cooled down, it's a concentrate prepared by steeping ground coffee in room temperature water for over twelve hours, which can be then served hot or cold. The intensity of the brew depends on several factors—the time, amount and temperature of water used and whether the coffee grounds are medium or coarse—but most aficionados say cold brew is smoother in texture. It's certainly lower in caffeine levels and is less acidic (it has a pH of 6.3 compared to a pH of 5.5 for hot brew).

Alcohol: A controversial subject, but experts tend to agree that moderate drinking (one or two drinks, two or three times a week) can protect us against heart disease and strokes. The kind of alcohol also matters. For instance, red wine contains powerful antioxidants that fight inflammation—but its benefits accrue when you do not consume more than a glass or two.

If you have a leaky gut, alcohol tolerance is significantly reduced and drinking it can injure the gut lining and promote or worsen inflammation. The clear message is that there is no single, 'safe' level of drinking. But since alcohol consumption cuts across cultures and is unlikely to disappear from our behaviour, what you can do to get the benefits of moderate drinking is to first heal the gut. And to drink alcohol in measured quantities. Binge drinking can never be good for your gut!

4 Fs: Fairly Fundamental

The four Fs are strong supportive adjuncts in your diet that you should adopt in your dietary journey to good health.

Functional Foods: These are foods that offer health benefits beyond their inherent nutritional value. They are protective foods and derive their goodness from non-nutrient compounds like phytonutrients, fibre and enzymes as well as pro- and prebiotics. Examples are garlic and onions (allyl sulfides in them help prevent heart disease); flaxseeds (lignans in them protect against cancer); and cabbage, cauliflower and broccoli (they contain indoles and isothiocyanates that offer protection from cancer). The probiotics in fermented dairy products and the prebiotics in whole grains and garlic aid gut function and improve immunity.

Sprouts are powerhouses as well. The germination process multiplies the nutrients, manufacturing vitamins and enzymes that weren't there originally. For instance, grains, seeds and pulses do not contain much vitamin C, but sprouting increases the vitamin C content by over 50 per cent and the vitamin B content by 20–30 per cent. Sprouting also destroys most of the common inhibitors present in grains and pulses (tannins, phytates, etc.) that bind to iron and calcium and interfere with their absorption. Sprouting in beans breaks down carbohydrates that cause gas. Alfalfa sprouts contain saponins, which lower bad cholesterol.

FOSHU (foods for specified health use) is a Japanese categorization for foods proven effective in maintaining health, which also meet safety standards. There are about 1200 FOSHU foods. Indians have traditionally known the wisdom of consuming functional foods, and we would benefit from a similar regulatory standards system.

Fermented Foods: Cultured dairy products (dahi, chhachh, etc.) contain probiotics or good bacteria that aid the gut. They also increase the production of butyrate, which helps gut health. Other fermented foods, such as vegetable kanjis, rice congee, kombucha, kimchi, kefir and sauerkraut, also contain 'live' microorganisms that promote enhanced digestion. They are a sub-category of functional foods but can be given their own heading, so useful are they in providing digestive support. Fermentation also allows beneficial bacteria to digest and degrade some lectins present in food. That's why foods such as idli, dosa, dhokla, sourdough bread, sauerkraut, kefir and yogurt are easy to digest for most people.

Fresh: Eating fresh has a two-pronged reference: first, it means using ingredients that are freshly grown and harvested, rather than those that come from a cold store or a freezer. Freshly picked vegetables have a high concentration of nutrients.

Second, it's also about cooking quantities according to how much you want to consume in a particular meal. Keeping cooked food in a refrigerator or for long periods in the freezer is not the ideal option, though it may be necessary sometimes. Refrigerator and stored food can increase histamine in foods and irritate the gut in people who are histamine-intolerant or have a sensitive gut. Buying fresh, wholesome produce and cooking meal-sized portions is better than living on leftovers. It enhances nutritional value and lowers the risk of infection.

Fasting: The concept of fasting has always been known in India; in fact, you will notice that almost every religion has fasting as part of its practices. The reason is that fasting is a useful detox and reset mechanism, and this knowledge has been present through the generations.

More recently, the idea of **Intermittent Fasting** has taken health enthusiasts by storm. This concept breaks away from earlier theories of small, frequent meals and that of breakfast being the biggest meal of the day—and says you should eat only within an eight-hour period. And starve the body for the other sixteen hours.

This is modern packaging of something the ancients knew already: fasting can actually protect the gut microbiome and the immune system. How does fasting work? Not eating for ten to twelve hours tends to starve the bacteria in the gut, but it starves bad bacteria more than good bacteria, so it improves gut flora balance. Fasting also helps the body's clean-up process and improves the immune function performed by the lining of the intestine. It's rest for the gut. Dr Yoshinori Ohsumi won the 2016 Nobel Prize for Medicine for his research on autophagy (the process during which cells break down and get rid of damaged structures, toxins, bacteria and viruses). Ohsumi discovered that fasting for long hours triggers the process of autophagy, which is critical for cell renewal.

Also, there are no advantages if the fasting is followed by feasting. Eating unhealthy fried vegetables and grains (kuttu-coated fried pakoras) or sugar-loaded sweets, as happens in many religious fasts, does not provide any gut gain.

SIRTUINS: THE POWER GENES

- Sirtuins are housekeeping genes, which are responsible for the repair and maintenance of cells.
- We all have these 'skinny genes'. In mammals, there are seven of them. They determine our ability to burn fat and our susceptibility to disease, and help regulate our lifespans.
- Recent studies in which yeast cells were engineered to produce higher than normal levels of sirtuins made the cells live 30 per cent longer.
- What gives sirtuins this power? Their ability to make cells switch to a survival mode, in which cellular toxins are cleared and fat is burnt.
- How can we activate sirtuins? Fasting, exercise and certain foods.
- Plant chemicals called polyphenols can help activate sirtuins.
- Nutritionists are working on a 'sirtfood' diet: it is high in plant-based foods that contain polyphenols and sirtuin activators (berries, turmeric, kale, coffee, chocolate, red onions, extra virgin olive oil, etc.).

Chapter XI

The Third P

'A goal without a plan is just a wish'
—Antoine de Saint-Exupéry

Failing to recognize the importance of planning meals, mealtimes, exercise and supplements ahead of time is surely the biggest barrier to reaching your health goals in hectic, fast-paced lifestyles.

Just as we plan our meetings, travel and work, this is equally important. Often I hear clients saying that they got nothing to eat, and hence ate the wrong things, to which my response is 'You should have planned and anticipated!'

P3. Planning: The principles of planning your meals are as important as knowing what to choose. Planning means working out **when** to eat the foods that work for you, as meal timing plays a critical role in determining health outcomes. Plan meals in conformity with both chrono nutrition and your personal requirements (what your goals are, by measuring your BMI, waist size and the location of fat on your body).

Chrono Nutrition refers to coordinating your food intake with the body's diurnal (also called circadian) rhythms. The body functions according to several internal checks and balances, which are synchronized with both its internal rhythm and those of nature (day and night; seasonal changes). Harmony with circadian rhythms has been demonstrated when evaluating indices like core temperature, cardio and respiratory function, brain activity, coagulation and immunity, to name a few.

Internally, when one organ is at peak performance level and energy, the organ that is on the opposite side of the clock is at its lowest level; research suggests that when the liver is at its peak between 1 and 3 a.m., cleansing the blood, the small intestine is at its lowest.

What does this mean? Since the intestine helps in the absorption and assimilation of nutrients, eating late at night is heavy on the digestive system. If you eat late, the food is poorly digested and absorbed—and the liver doesn't get time to do its housekeeping and clean-up job properly. The body is not programmed to function well if there is late-night socializing, drinking and eating.

Studies suggest that eating against the biological clock increases inflammatory markers as well. It is therefore not surprising that night shift work is called the 'graveyard shift'! Those who work late nights are at higher risk of having heart attacks and strokes.[1]

THE ORGAN CLOCK

Lungs: work best in the early morning. Cardio activity should be scheduled early in the day.

Gut: the large colon's preferred time to cleanse is in the morning.

Stomach/Pancreas/Small Intestine: all prefer heavier meals earlier in the day; the stomach peaks in the morning, so breakfast is important. The small intestine would like heavier meals in the first half of the day.

Liver: this is the main detox organ of the body. It wants the last meal of the day consumed by the early evening so that it can cleanse at its high energy time, in the wee hours of the night.

For chrono nutrition, you also need to see what your day involves, your work, your exercise routine and when you feel most hungry in order to decide the timing of your most substantial meal. For some, that could be lunch, for others an early dinner. Some people need a big breakfast, others a big dinner. Once you work out when your peak meal time is, that's the time you should eat the maximum quantity of grains or cereal.

Observational studies suggest that most people peak either at lunch or between 5 and 7 p.m. Whenever you decide to eat the main grain-heavy meal, dietary wisdom

lies in completing this before 7 p.m. Even if your dinner
is the light meal, do finish it by 7 p.m. Anyone who is
still hungry later, after eating a substantial meal before
7 p.m., can supplement it with soup, salad, fruits, nuts
or protein later, to ward off hunger pangs. Clear herbal
teas, hot chocolate and liquids also help calm hunger
signals at night.

A.M. AND P.M.

4 a.m. to noon: Elimination of waste
Noon to 8 p.m.: Appropriation of food (eating and
digestion)
8 p.m. to 4 a.m.: Assimilation and use; the cleaning
crew comes in the latter half of this period

Be a Diarist: In order to coordinate these
fundamentals of what, how much and when to eat,
you need to keep a record of whatever you eat. Keep
a food diary or journal. Research shows that most
people underestimate what they eat and overestimate
how much they exercise. Many of those who consult
me for weight loss report eating very small quantities
of carbohydrates. Keeping a detailed food diary acts as
a reality check and stops the denial.

A food journal is an important tool because it
takes consumption away from the subjective (what
you think you eat) to the objective (what you actually
consume). It will also show how balanced your diet is,
particularly in terms of fruits and vegetables, nuts and

seeds, etc. You should also write down how you feel after consuming most foods.

Soon, patterns will emerge. If you experience bloating, acidity, diarrhoea or flatulence after a particular food or a combination of foods, that is a clue to your sensitivities or intolerances. The food diary helps create a reference point that helps you design a dietary strategy that works **FOR YOU**. Customize your plan to fit your work pattern, your social life and definitely, your most-loved cheat foods. Because we should sin occasionally. The thumb rule is to cheat with what you absolutely love and not just for the heck of it. If you write it down, you will know how often you do so—and the effect it has.

You can use the food diary to plan the rule-breaking too. Select the better of the unhealthy food cravings that you might have, or just eat a smaller quantity. **Less** truly is **More!** But by no means should you cheat on the foods you are sensitive to. That will destroy all the good work you have done healing the gut.

PSST

PSST is an acronym for foods you are better off without or those you should ingest in very small quantities. PSST stands for **Processed food, Salt, Sugar and Trans fats**.

Avoid These

Processed Foods: Diets rich in processed or junk food are double trouble for the body; they result in weight gain and also have a poor status in nutrition. Such foods are also high in high-fructose corn syrup, additives and hidden sugars—all of which have an adverse impact on the gut. People who eat processed foods regularly tend to be at risk of nutritional deficiencies and this can activate the autoimmunity disorder switch.

Salt: We need salt for flavour, and a certain level of sodium is necessary for the body to maintain fluid balance and transmit nerve impulses. But how much salt is good for you? The answer: not very much.

The recommended salt intake is no more than 6 gm a day—that is about 1 teaspoon. If you consume more than that, it attracts water, so the blood volume increases. This raises blood pressure since the heart has to work harder to maintain pressure in the arteries. The higher your blood pressure, the greater the strain on your heart, arteries, kidneys and brain. This can increase the risk of heart attacks, strokes, dementia and kidney disease.

Which foods are high in salt? Processed foods (pizzas, bread, cold cuts, sausages, bacon, cheese) are usually high in salt and additives that contain sodium. All vegetables, dairy products, meat and shellfish are natural sources of sodium. Some condiments too are sodium-rich—for instance, a tablespoon of soy sauce contains 1000 mg of sodium. Mustard, sauces, pickles, chutneys and dressings are high in salt content too, so limit their intake. Freshly cooked meats and vegetables, seasoned with fresh herbs and spices and just a little salt, are the ideal way to get the right daily dose of salt.

Sugar: Detailed in Chapter V, I just want to remind you that you can get plenty of sugar from starchy veggies or from natural sources such as honey and jaggery, and from fruit. Processed sugar (the white sugar that's added to tea, coffee, soft drinks, desserts and sauces) is a refined carbohydrate. Sugars contain empty calories, with little or no nutrient value. Eating food with sugar may give you a temporary energy boost but it promotes insulin resistance and weight gain. Worse, you should know that many foods that are advertised as low-fat are high in sugar content (examples are breakfast cereals and low-fat granola). In fact, such foods can raise blood cholesterol levels. And high sugar intake changes the gut flora balance—negatively.

Trans fats: Trans-fatty acids, or TFAs, are fats that should be strictly avoided. These are manmade fats that are not recognized by the body. They occur when vegetable oils are chemically altered (usually hydrogenated) to stay solid at room temperature. Many people start the day with just these fats—they are used in manufacturing many kinds of biscuits and rusks—with your morning cup of tea. One of my biggest challenges is to get clients to agree to not eat biscuits, namkeens and other fried snacks—they contain trans fats and refined flour and are combined with sugar or salt.

Trans fats have been linked to the development of cardiovascular disease; they increase blood cholesterol levels, reduce HDL or good cholesterol and increase the risk of clotting. In India, there are regulations that food manufacturers who use fat must declare the trans-fat content on their labels. So, carefully read the information on processed food products. TFAs cause 5 lakh deaths worldwide annually. Indians eating out get 30–40 per cent TFAs, whereas their content should be no more than 1 per cent of the total calories consumed.

Apart from trans fats, refined vegetable oils are also fat offenders, because refined oil has to be stabilized and the high temperatures at which this occurs destroy most of the antioxidants and essential fatty acids present in them. They also contain other additives to make them chemically stable. Excess intake of refined oils high in polyunsaturated fatty acids (PUFA) can be inflammatory to the system.

In fact, refined vegetable oils replaced conventional, traditional fats used in homes as well as in commercial food production, for example, desi ghee, butter, mustard oil and sesame oil were replaced by refined sunflower, kardi, corn, soya oils, vanaspati and margarine. Ironically, the science behind this changeover was based on several studies suggesting that saturated fats and cholesterol were causing heart disease. The facts were not as simple and, in the bargain, we neither stopped the epidemic nor understood the collateral damage that happens because of this. We ended up losing our highly nutritious traditional fats and began using chemical-laden unstable oils and inflammatory molecules, such as trans fats. The vegetable oils are being frequently used now; sunflower, safflower, corn and soyabean oils are not only high heat-refined—thereby losing their goodness—but also high in pro-inflammatory polyunsaturated fats.

And then there is **frying**, a process that makes many foods delicious (who doesn't relish puris or pakoras?). Frying food, however, creates a triple whammy: it increases the fat content; reduces the nutritional content by destroying the vitamins and affecting the proteins adversely; and the chemical changes to the oils themselves are harmful ones. Intense heating can change natural fats in the oils to trans fats, which have unfavourable health outcomes (see the write-up on fats in Chapter X). The high heat also releases volatile decomposition products (VDP) that stay in the leftover oil and if it is reused, get into the food. This irritates the gut lining. Extended heating also forms harmful chemicals in the oil, such as acrolein, a cancer-causing compound.

What Should You Do to Make Frying Healthier?

- Minimize frying.
- Fry at a moderate 200-degree temperature and pan-fry briefly. When the temperature is too low, the food absorbs more oil; when it is too high, the outside may brown while the food item stays raw inside.
- Don't reheat the oil used for frying. It is best to use a minimal quantity and discard the oil after the first use, but if this is not economical, strain all the burnt particles from it and store it in a refrigerator. Reuse it quickly.

SNACKS: NO THANKS

- *Chai* and *samosa*? That staple snack of the Indian office is just about the worst thing that we can consume, particularly in a sedentary job. If you have an office canteen, scan the menu; it's like a list of the worst possible food combinations: cheese toast, bread pakoras, samosas, pizzas, etc. They are rich in trans fats, salt and hidden sugars.
- Soft drinks are anything but soft on your system, as they contain vast amounts of sugar.
- Saying no to heavy snacks at work or at home at the witching (read teatime) hour is your best dietary present to yourself.
- Most people oscillate between being either snackers or the kind who skip meals and then binge eat. Neither of these eating patterns is good for you.
- Poor eating habits, added to the stress of one's work environment, lead to lifestyle disorders

Equally Essential Elements

These are the principles that provide structure and strategy along the road to good health. They are the acronyms **BLES**, **SLO** and **EDSS**. You also need to develop the art of **managing stress** to keep the journey smooth and practise the life skills outlined in **YAMS**.

BLES Yourself

This is a simple acronym for *how* to eat. It stands for the common-sense dietary wisdom of:

- Eat **Better**
- Eat **Less**
- Eat **Early** and
- Eat **Slowly** (chew well).

Eating Better is about choosing foods that have high nutrient density, right from fruits and vegetables to whole grains and proteins. In fact, these need not be low-calorie—coconut, avocado, nuts and their oils and seeds score high on the calorie scale—but what is important is that they are loaded with nutrients, vitamins and minerals. Many such foods also possess high satiation levels, so they can keep you from eating too much. Eggs, for example, are a food that's packed with nutrients, but relatively low in calories. Basically, the approach should be to pick high-value foods (that are full of nutrients) and not really count calories.

That brings us to the next point: **Eat Less**. Choose quality over quantity; your gut will thank you for it. Contrary to what most people believe, consuming a smaller amount of high-nutrient-value foods will not lower your energy levels, it will raise them! All my clients are surprised to see how small their appetites become when they begin their dietary journey with me—yet they have phenomenal levels of energy. Their sleep requirements go down and fatigue becomes history!

Overeating has both short-term and long-term effects—none of them good. It increases appetite and puts pressure to produce more enzymes. The body's capacity to generate digestive juices is finite; frequent overeating means consistently slowed digestion and digestive disorders such as heartburn from the extra acid produced. In the long term, the food is more likely to be stored as fat. In fact, several studies as well as an analysis of the diet of the centenarian communities show that low-calorie diets are associated with longevity and lower risk of disease. Restricting calories decreases atherosclerosis and free radicals and improves insulin sensitivity. These are all markers of longevity.

Portion control begins at the serving stage. Put less on the plate. Or, put all that you want at one time, rather than going for seconds. Looking at a full plate also increases fullness—quite literally! We also eat with our eyes!

Tip: Follow the Japanese saying, 'Hara Hachi Bu', the practice of eating until you feel 80 per cent full. It is believed to be the secret of the centenarian Japanese. Among north Indians, it's said that you should leave place for one roti when you finish a meal. As our ancestors would put it:

Ek kaal bhoji, Yogi (one who eats one meal a day is one whose wants are controlled)

Dwi kaal bhoji, Bhogi (one who eats two meals a day is one who wants to enjoy everything)

Tri kaal bhoji, Rogi! (one who eats three meals a day is someone who is often ill)

Words of wisdom we have buried under the weight of modern lifestyles!

Eat Early, giving your gut the time to break down the food you eat in the most efficient manner possible. This will not just provide a healthy amount of nutrition but giving a good gap between a meal and bedtime will help you sleep better. As I have said before, the timing of meals is critical to good health. Eat between the hours of 7 a.m. and 7 p.m., according to the natural circadian rhythm of day and night. In other words, 'Eat during the working hours of your system!'

Eating Slowly has a number of benefits. First, the digestive process actually starts in the mouth, so chewing slowly and chewing well improves digestion. Second, it gives the gut the time (about twenty minutes) it needs to register satiation levels. Hunger hormones get suppressed and the 'I'm full' message gets released, which helps you stop eating before you overeat.

Dial it Down

SLO: The logic of the acronym **SLO** is unassailable. First, eat foods that are **seasonal**. Items that are out of season, such as strawberries in summer in India that are flown in or transported by road from far (reducing freshness) or brought out from cold stores. Not only are they lower in nutrients but it's also quite likely that these items have been sprayed with preservatives or chemicals to improve storage and transport. The best option is to go for the cheapest fruits and vegetables. They are likely to be seasonal.

Eat Local: Locally grown foods aren't just fresh. They have the geographic benefit of being suited to the climate in the region where they are being consumed. For instance, there is a reason why lauki, tori and kakdi are available in large quantities in the hot summer months in north India. They are rich in water content and nutrients. Ditto with summer fruit: melons, watermelons, peaches, plums and the like. Gourd vegetables are also light in calorie content, so are good for summer menus.

Eat Organic: One cannot stress the importance of shifting to the consumption of organically grown fruits and vegetables, grains and pulses. As I explained in the chapter on the thirty-five Ps, commercially-grown food products are often sprayed with pesticides and the soils they are grown in have fertilizer and chemicals added to improve yield and avoid pests. Organic crops are grown without the use of fertilizers and pesticides, so they do not contain the residue from these chemicals. The added advantage of more microbes in the soil is that there are more minerals in the grains and pulses as well.

Nifty Tools

The acronym **EDSS** refers to some useful tools that you should learn to employ along this dietary journey.

Elimination: I have said this before but, armed with all the information until now, you can use the tool of elimination wisely, to cut out foods that you might be sensitive to. If you do not respond to whatever changes you have made in your diet and lifestyle, you may be suffering from a food sensitivity. As a thumb rule, begin by eliminating inflammatory grains such as wheat, barley, oats and rye. If that doesn't help resolve issues, look at dairy and so on.

Diary: That all-important journal in which you write literally 'everything' you eat, when you eat it, how often—and how you feel once you have consumed it.

Seek: Never be afraid of consulting a health professional. To understand what your testing protocol reveals or if you see a change in the parameters, seek out a nutritionist or doctor. Test results, especially food sensitivity tests, can be often overwhelming and need interpretation.

Supplement: You cannot always get everything you need from food alone; sometimes, that can be because your leaky gut has to first heal before you can absorb essential nutrients, or sometimes it can be because your personal beliefs lead you to avoid certain foods or because you are intolerant to gluten or dairy. You may then need to add certain supplements that will not just address deficiencies but help the intestines heal, so that nutrients are better absorbed.

FOOD SYSTEM: THE BIG PICTURE

Safe and _Swachh_: Food must be safe, microbially, and free from adulteration or toxins

Sustainable: The food system must address good agricultural practices, diets and food waste management

Sufficient: Everyone should get an adequate amount and distribution should be equitable

And Lastly, Some Vital Life Skills

Stress Management: Stress is not just a feeling. The gut–brain connection is an intimate one and it works both ways: a troubled intestine can send signals to the brain and vice versa. Mental stress can and does cause intestinal distress. And don't we all know this? The rush to the bathroom when tension mounts is the simplest way to understand this connection.

This occurs because stress causes a biochemical reaction by releasing a hormone called cortisol into the bloodstream. High levels of cortisol create inflammation in the gut. It can lead to gastrointestinal disorders. Chronic stress and chronic inflammation can lead to diseases like hypertension, cardiac disease, cancer and almost all digestive diseases.

Dietary change can help manage stress and begin a process of healing in the gut but there are some useful techniques that calm the gut and press the reset button on your health. I've called them **YAMS.**

Yoga: It doesn't have to specifically be yoga. A regular exercise regimen will do—the accent is on the regular. Yoga, though, is a proven centuries-old science that uses virtually all the muscles of the body and even has asanas dedicated to digestion! Yoga, as the name suggests (*yog* or union), is a practice that helps the individual attain a union between the physical, mental and spiritual aspects of his or her being. It consists of a holistic and regular practice of physical postures (asanas), breath control techniques (pranayama) and deep relaxation and meditation. It brings harmony within and energizes all the elements of good health.

The asanas relax and rejuvenate the body while keeping the mind active, yet calm. The method ensures that the body is relaxed but the nerves that connect the body extend, expand and relax; this naturally quietens the mind. The asanas are practised with regulating the flow of breath, helping it become smooth and quiet, thereby calming the stressed mind. They do not rush the muscles but keep them active and alert without strain. Regular practice of yoga brings a transformational change in the physical, mental and emotional state of an individual, all with a positive impact. Yoga never tires you; it refreshes you!

Scientific studies have also found that recitation of yoga mantras (sutras from the scriptures) benefits both the mind and the body. Only a calm mind and body can boost its immunity. Thus, yoga helps boost the immune system and, when combined with a light diet, the practice of yoga can help reverse lifestyle diseases, and improve sleep and digestion. And make the body stronger to resist infection.

Aerobic: Aerobic means that the body uses oxygen to produce energy for exercise. Such exercise can improve circulation, cardiovascular, digestive and immune system function and lower the risk of developing heart disease. To derive maximum benefit, exercise for thirty to forty-five minutes, three to five times a week. Examples of aerobic exercises are:

- brisk walking, jogging, skipping or cycling
- treadmill, cross-trainer, Zumba, Pilates, kickboxing
- swimming, badminton, tennis or squash

For those who have had mainly sedentary lives until now, bring in a change:

- Begin walking; climb flights of stairs; avoid the lift
- Park a little further away and walk part of the way

Remember to increase your stamina by slow but steady increments in pace and distance. Work out according to a target heart rate zone, calculated by subtracting your age from 220 and multiplying the result by the percentage you want to achieve. The optimum level is between 50 and 75 per cent.

Our ancient yogis knew that just the rapid breathing techniques in pranayama help improve oxygen saturation levels in the blood by exercising the diaphragm. They also help reduce blood pressure. Pranayama works in conjunction with yoga and meditation to activate the parasympathetic system through the vagus nerve to reduce stress and increase inner calm, both in the mind and in the gut.

Meditation: Although we must eat right to keep the gut healthy, our state of mind is also crucial to maintain gut flora balance.

The body's autonomous nervous system, which controls the fight-flight response, consists of the sympathetic system (the body engine's accelerator, the 'fight or flight' response) and the parasympathetic system (the 'rest and digest' response).

In a host with chronic stress, the sympathetic system is constantly active; this impairs digestion. The parasympathetic system is the brake, the relax response. Your body needs both the accelerator and the brake to be in optimum working order; only then will the engine hum along in harmony.

Meditation slows the frantic activity of the sympathetic system and increases that of the parasympathetic. As it calms the mind, it also calms the gut. This can reduce inflammation in the body, help heal a leaky gut and maintain a healthy gut barrier for the future. It also improves nutrient absorption and metabolism.

Sleep: The condition of your gut microbiome and the quality of your sleep are closely related. A study by researchers at Nova Southwestern University[2] found that subjects who slept well had better gut flora diversity than those with poor sleep patterns. Dr Jaime Tartar, a research director of the study, says that the deepest stage of sleep is when the brain 'takes out the trash'. A good night's sleep basically flushes out the byproducts of neural activity that accumulate during the waking hours. Good sleep is critical, therefore, to good housekeeping of the body.

In another study,[3] researchers at Rochester University discovered that the brain has its own unique waste removal system; just as the lymphatic system removes cellular waste from the body, the brain has its own closed circuit system (dubbed the glymphatic system), which is active during the hours we are asleep, and it clears the toxins responsible for neurological disorders.

Melatonin is a master hormone, secreted by the pineal gland, that plays an important role in setting the body's twenty-four-hour clock. It helps regulate waking and sleep patterns, and protects the body from ageing and even from some cancers. It's stimulated by darkness and its release is blocked by light. The pineal gland begins secreting it in the evening, and it peaks at about midnight. When melatonin levels are high, you feel drowsy. The production of melatonin reduces with age, and for some, supplements might be prescribed.

RELAXATION TECHNIQUES: CREATING CALM

- Find a quiet spot.
- Close your eyes and breathe slowly, counting the breaths down from five to one.
- Then, focus on your breathing and try to relax.

- Imagine yourself in a calm, light place and focus on that or focus on a particular mantra.
- You can listen to a relaxation tape.
- Practise diaphragmatic breathing:
  - ◆ Sit in a comfortable position
  - ◆ Place your hands under the ribs, with the fingers pointing towards the belly
  - ◆ Inhale slowly through the nose: the fingertips should feel the ribs moving to the side
  - ◆ Exhale through the mouth: with each outward breath, allow tension to leave the body, and relaxation to enter

Sleep hygiene is a term that refers to the practices that help produce better sleep. They include avoiding stimulants like caffeine, excess alcohol and heavy meals close to bedtime. Regular exercise and exposure to natural light are important too. A warm water bath and stopping screen time a couple of hours before getting into bed can significantly improve the quantity and quality of sleep. Reading, listening to calming music or meditation helps as well.

The quality of your sleep impacts many other facets of health. Sleep deprivation can negatively impact the body's sugar control. The result can be insulin sensitivity, increased appetite and the accumulation of visceral fat. A sound sleep keeps the gut calm and a calm gut protects the body from inflammation. Shakespeare was right: sleep indeed *'knits up the ravell'd sleave of care'*!

Important Note

While the 4 Rs protocol (as explained in Chapter IX) has been presented as a step-wise approach, this is simply an explanatory device. In actual fact, you will be working on multiple phases at the same time. For example, removing irritating foods, compounds and pathogens from the digestive tract is the first step, but beginning this process also automatically initiates the body's own repair mechanisms. And most of the techniques and tools required to implement the rules have to be undertaken together; all the directive principles need to be applied, to begin well and continue on the journey to dietary health.

Most importantly, if you're getting only six hours of sleep (or less) a night, your gut-healing diet can only take you so far. Or if you are stressed at work or at home, and not able to manage it, the resultant release of cortisol will create inflammation in the gut.

The best practice is: internalize these rules and principles comprehensively, use them to make transformational changes to your dietary habits and then chart a steady course towards health. Good intent makes good intestines, but good intestines can and will metamorphose intentions into good health!

TEN HABITS FOR HAPPINESS

1. Attitude
2. Diet
3. Destress
4. Contentment
5. Giving Back
6. Movement
7. Purpose
8. Relationships
9. Sleep
10. Spirituality

Chapter XII

Immunity: A Formidable Weapon

It's 2022 and since spring 2020, much of the world's population has experienced lockdowns and social restrictions or has been advised to stay home as much as possible. Everyone has been recommended the twin preventive practices of social distancing and consistent hygiene to guard against contracting the diabolical coronavirus that has ravaged millions of lives across the globe. Over the last few months, however, we have also had to come to terms with the fact that this and perhaps other pathogens are here for the long term. And that we do have to step out and perform regular and essential activities under its cloud of lurking danger.

COVID-19 is like an unwanted guest—it is here to stay! Even now, there is little chance that it will disappear completely from the world any time soon. The virus also doesn't respect any borders (of districts, states or countries). It dictates the timeline of its activity and virulence. We are really not in control of the virus—*who* will get infected, with *what* symptoms (or asymptomatic) and with *what* outcomes?

Is it purely a game of chance, a horrible Russian Roulette? Not quite. This virus, like every other pathogen, is actively seeking a host; what we **can** do is to make our bodies less hospitable, to not open the doors and windows of our body to let it in and take hold.

The barrier that we have in our control, apart from masking, distancing and hygiene, is a strong immune system, the body's own defence mechanism against external threats. Immunity is the best weapon you have to minimize the chances of getting infected if exposed—or of fighting off an infection successfully.

How does one boost immunity?

Understanding Immunity

Before we address the issue of building immunity, let's briefly understand what this term means and how the immune system works.

Immunity is the hallmark of the immune system, an elaborate and finely-tuned defence system that works to destroy and counter the effects of disease-causing viruses, bacteria, yeasts and other foreign substances that operate within tissues, cells in the bloodstream and the lymph.

There are some terms associated with immunity that we should understand: innate and adaptive (acquired) immunity, and humoral and cell-mediated immunity.

Innate: This is the immunity we are born with; even newborn babies have an ingrained immunity that recognizes foreign bodies and reacts to their presence.

Adaptive: The adaptive immune system differentiates between what is part of the body and what is foreign and is programmed to react to what it sees as alien. In any human body, the interplay between innate and adaptive immunity creates a dynamic situation in which inflammation is the reaction to foreign substances. If the body's defences are unable to completely eliminate the alien pathogen, it results in infection (as can happen in COVID-19). The adaptive immunity of the body can be naturally acquired by contact with a pathogen (like influenza or COVID-19) or artificially, through vaccinations, etc.

See Fig. 4 below for a break-up.

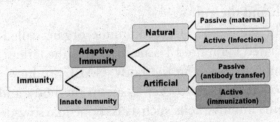

Fig. 4

The body's adaptive immunity can also be divided by the kind of immune mediators, into humoral immunity and cell-mediated immunity.

Humoral Immunity: It involves substances found in body fluids, also called humours (e.g., blood and lymph) and is mediated by antibodies.

Cell-Mediated Immunity: This is the other component of adaptive immunity within the cell and is mediated by activated, antigen-specific T cells and cytokines. One of the problems with COVID-19 is that it over-stimulates the production of cytokines, creating a cytokine storm that threatens to overwhelm the body. Cytokines (proteins or peptides) are produced by specific immune cells (T-helper cells, lymphocytes) in response to an antigen (pathogen) and help in the defence system.

Unlike other systems in the body, which consist of a definite set of organs—for example, the nervous system is made up of the brain, the spinal cord and the nerves, or the urinary system has a pair of kidneys, the ureter and the bladder—the immune system operates through several sites in the body, including the spleen, liver, the spinal cord, the brain and connective tissue, the skin, blood, bone marrow, the thymus gland, the lymph and **the gut**.

The gut is the largest immune organ, called Gut-Associated Lymphoid Tissue or GALT, the largest mass of lymphoid tissue in the body. GALT produces more antibodies than any other tissue in the body and also contains immune cells such as B (bone marrow-derived lymphocytes) and T lymphocytes (or thymus-derived lymphocytes, produced in the bone marrow), most famously called T cells. Research suggests that 70–80 per cent of your immune system is in your gut.

It is, therefore, logical to note that any disturbance in the gut can trigger an abnormal immune response in the body. It is, also, not surprising then, that diseases of the immune system, such as autoimmune disorders, cancers, arthritis, etc., have increased exponentially with a rise in gut-related issues.

Enter COVID-19. This virus and its arc of infection have thrown up unexpected and unusual demands from our immune system. Strengthening the immune system of your body means that the gut, which is the frontline of this potential battle, must be healed. If you have a leaky gut, it creates inflammation and this weakens your immunity.

So, it's quite clear that the foundation of a healthy immune system lies in the digestive system being nurtured by diet and lifestyle. The gut is Ground Zero for immune defence. Immunity can be strengthened with nutrition, and our diet and food are the best vehicles.

In other words, though the coronavirus may attack your lungs and respiratory tract—**your defence against it begins in the GUT!**

THE SPECTRE OF COVID-19

- Rather like the larger-than-life villains in James Bond movies, SARS COVID-19 is a virulent pathogen.
- When we think of COVID-19, we think of people with cough and pneumonia, struggling to breathe, being put on ventilators.
- But the ACE2 receptors this virus attacks are not just present in our lungs—they are also in the gastrointestinal tract.
- That's why the composition of your gut microbiome is a critical component of how a host body responds to COVID-19.

Immunity, as I have explained in this book, is mediated through the microbiome, the vast host of microbes that dwell in the gut. Two-thirds of the body's immune system is in the gut. Among these trillions of microbes, there are good and bad microbes, and as anyone who has ever balanced their accounts knows, it's obvious that our immunity balance should lean in favour of good microbes instead of those that are inimical to us. If we feed our microbes what they like, they work in our favour; if we give them food they dislike, they work against us. The road to better immunity starts with better nutrition.

Nutrition That Benefits the Immune System

The immune system requires an array of nutrients, including proteins, fatty acids, vitamins and minerals to function well. Poor dietary choices can lead to both malnutrition (low in minerals and vitamins) and over-nutrition (high in calories, salt, sugar and toxic fats). These weaken the immune system. Malnourished individuals who lack adequate nutrients through good calories are prone to disease. Chronic deficiencies of nutrients lower immunity. Supplements are often needed due to malabsorption caused by a leaky gut, or among the elderly or those who are immunocompromised (this can include chronic dieters). Supplements are also needed when we use nutrients like vitamins and minerals as therapeutic agents or detoxifiers: Vitamin C, B vitamins, vitamin D and zinc are required in higher amounts to protect the body in the wake of an epidemic, stress or pollution. Requirements are also high in people who smoke or drink alcohol or have a poor nutritional status for other reasons.

A recent study published on the preprint server *medRxiv*[1] in May 2020 shows that a combination of the readily available and inexpensive vitamins D3, B12, and the mineral magnesium can reduce the progression of COVID-19 to severe or fatal stages.

Antioxidant Benefit

To do this effectively, your diet should be varied, with a strong emphasis on whole foods, fruits and vegetables, especially those rich in vitamin C, beta carotene and other carotenoids (plant version of vitamin A). Supplementing your food with 100 per cent of the RDA (recommended daily allowance) of B vitamins and trace minerals, such as zinc and magnesium, is a prudent form of insurance. And if your food intake is 1600 calories or less, or contains junk food, this supplementation is essential.

Antioxidant nutrients such as vitamins and minerals enhance immune responses by lowering the burden of free radicals (unstable and reactive atoms, which are associated with disease and ageing). They thus protect immune cells against cumulative oxidation and free radical attack due to the release of powerful oxidizing agents such as superoxide, hydrogen peroxide and hydroxyl radicals.

Vitamins

Vitamin C: You've all heard that taking vitamin C helps ward off a cold. The reason: this vitamin plays an integral role in boosting immunity. Taking vitamin C increases antioxidants in the blood by as much as 30 per cent, and this strengthens the body's defences in fighting inflammation. A deficiency of vitamin C lowers the immune response in animal models; adequate vitamin C increases the production of T and B cells (cells used to destroy pathogens) and helps attacking cells migrate to sites of infection while making viruses and bacteria more sensitive to destruction.

Our bodies cannot manufacture vitamin C; we must get it from food sources or supplements. It's found in citrus fruits, guavas and vegetables such as spinach. Amla or Indian gooseberry is the richest source of vitamin C. Ample vitamin C sources are available naturally, and they are often better than taking large doses of capsules.

Vitamin A and **Beta Carotene:** It was known as the eyesight vitamin but its immune boosting system function earned it the title 'the infection vitamin' in the early twentieth century. Vitamin A and beta carotene are needed for the integrity of the skin and the intestinal tract and they help maintain the thymus gland during stress. Overproduction of cortisol, a stress-induced hormone from the adrenal glands, tends to shrink the thymus gland, which is critical for fully-functioning T cells.

Limited studies suggest that beta carotene may also help stimulate helper T cells. Studies of children in developing nations indicate that there is a direct relationship between vitamin A deficiency and decreased resistance to infection. Excessive amounts of vitamin A, however, can decrease immune system function and can be toxic. Food sources include orange and yellow vegetables and fruits, as well as green leafy vegetables, butter and eggs.[2]

Vitamin D: Vitamin D, or the sunshine vitamin, doesn't just help our intestines absorb more calcium and magnesium but, like vitamin A, it is also integral in helping maintain the integrity of our gut lining, the membrane that forms a barrier between us and the environment. It's important to maintain optimum levels of vitamin D. Exposure to the sun helps in the synthesis of vitamin D, but this activity is hampered by high levels of pollutants in the air and supplements might be needed. Also, if there is an inflammation in the gut, it can compromise the metabolism of vitamin D, making us deficient. Food sources, though limited, include eggs, butter, fish oil and foods fortified with the vitamin.

B Vitamins: This refers to a group of eight vitamins, B5, B6, B12 and folic acid being among the common ones. **Folic Acid** helps the body produce and maintain new cells. It is required for immunity and lymphocyte protection. You can get folic acid from dried beans and peas or lentils, dark, leafy green vegetables, as well as broccoli and asparagus. Citrus is also an important source.

Vitamin B12 is important for the body to produce red blood cells and helps strengthen immunity. Animal proteins are rich in B12 and for vegetarians, fortified dairy products and fermented grains are good sources. A significant contribution of this vitamin comes from the gut microbiome, as the microbes produce it, but with an unhealthy gut, this process gets compromised.

Pantothenic Acid (Vitamin B5) and **Vitamin B6** help keep the lymphatic system and the thymus—a primary organ of the lymphatic system that lies behind the sternum bone in the upper chest, within which T cells mature—healthy. Foods such as mushrooms, avocados, eggs and lentils are good sources of vitamin B5. And sweet potatoes and bananas, apart from animal protein, can provide vitamin B6.

Vitamin E: It enhances both humoral and cell-mediated immunity because it involves antibodies. A deficiency of this vitamin contributes to a reduction in the functioning of T cells, killer cells and macrophages. Vitamin E supplements boost the immune system in older people who have a restricted diet, suggesting that older people require more vitamin E than specified in the adult RDA to ensure a fully functional immune system. Nuts, seeds, oils and eggs are good sources of vitamin E.

Minerals

Zinc helps maintain the lymph glands and the thymus, thereby helping to fight chronic infection. Zinc is also required for many important enzymes and it is not surprising that a deficiency of zinc decreases T cell and B cell function and macrophage activity. Zinc, in combination with trace minerals, including copper, iron and manganese, appears to improve B and T cell function in older people.

Zinc functions like an ionophore (a chemical species that binds ions). It transports zinc ions across a cell membrane and is associated with antiviral and anti-cancer activity. According to research, chloroquine, a zinc ionophore, quercetin, which is a catechin (found in apples, onions, grapes and berries), epigallocatechin gallate (found in green tea, tea, apples, avocados, berries and pistachios), all help transport zinc ions into cells and they block virus entry as well as prevent them from replicating. This is the hydroxychloroquine connection, the reason it was tried as a treatment for COVID-19 as well as given as a prophylactic to healthcare professionals.[3]

Magnesium: This is one of the most abundant minerals in the human body and is required in more than 300 metabolic functions. It helps activate phagocytes, which literally eat the foreign bodies. It's also required for antibody protection. Its deficiency is one of the most under-recognized; what makes it difficult is that it is not easily picked up by routine blood tests. Some common signs include poor brain function and memory issues, frequent headaches and migraines, digestive issues, heart function, blood pressure and insomnia (see box overleaf).

Food sources are bananas, avocados, coconut water, nuts, seeds, whole grains, beans, greens, vegetable juices, seafood, dark chocolate and rock salt (see the 'Sendha Namak' case on page 272). A leaky gut can affect the absorption of magnesium.

MAGNESIUM: THE MINERAL MARVEL

- The heart and other muscles rely on magnesium for proper contraction. Deficiency can cause racing heartbeats, slow ones or irregular rhythm. It can also disturb blood pressure.
- Insufficient magnesium is linked to insomnia and sleep issues.
- It regulates intestinal contractions, so can control bowel movements.
- Its deficiency is also related to muscle cramps and general body ache.
- Anxiety and mood disorders too can be activated by insufficient magnesium.
- Its role in the production of essential neurotransmitters means poor levels can result in imbalanced blood cholesterol, abdominal fat, high sugar levels, increased risk of strokes and seizures, peripheral neuropathy and more.
- And now, its role in post-COVID-19 recovery is also being considered.

Is magnesium a miracle pill? Not exactly, but it comes close. The benefits of adequate magnesium are quite extensive—it could help relax nerves and muscles, improve digestion and elimination and be a catalyst in improving health issues like diabetes, high blood pressure and heart disease.

COVID-19 Connection

The role of depleted magnesium because of infection could be a possible cause of sudden cardiac arrest among some patients who have recently recovered from COVID-19. Such depletion has also affected people who perform intense exercise and athletes. That physical exercise depletes the body of magnesium is a known fact (it is a water-soluble mineral, so you can sweat it out). But if intense exercise is combined with inadequate dietary intake of magnesium, or poor absorption because of inflammation or infection, it can severely affect energy metabolism and physical ability. Muscles need magnesium to function well and the heart muscle needs it too for proper contraction— there is a need for magnesium supplementation among those who are recovering from COVID-19 or any other major infection—and for those who are on long-term medication or who regularly perform very physical exercise.[4]

Selenium is a co-factor for an important antioxidant enzyme, glutathione peroxidase, which neutralizes lipid peroxidation, a process that can damage the immune cells. Selenium works with vitamin E to stimulate the immune response to infection in experimental animals. Together, they can help protect against cancer. Selenium increases helper T cells and increases antibody protection in experimental animals. However, excessive selenium depresses the immune system, so supplementation should only be under supervision. Sources of selenium are nuts, seeds, whole grains and eggs.

Iron is required to produce T and B cells: anaemia or iron deficiency is associated with an increased incidence of common infections among children. Iron deficiency can be because of insufficient consumption of the right kind of food or factors that help in its absorption. Food sources are green leafy vegetables, animal protein and black gram (kala chana). Pomegranate, beetroot and vitamin C enhance the absorption of iron. Cooking in cast iron vessels can improve the iron content of foods by as much as 300 per cent. A sprinkle of sesame seeds over vegetables and salads can also help.

A deficiency of **copper** is also associated with a higher risk of infection; copper deficiency diminishes the effectiveness of the humoral system in lab animals. Copper is an essential component of superoxide dismutase, an enzyme that helps break down oxygen molecules. Since it is involved in the absorption of iron, low copper levels can increase the risk of anaemia. Water stored in copper vessels along with food sources such as nuts, seeds and legumes is the best way to get dietary copper. Once again, excess levels can be toxic.

Manganese: A trace nutrient, manganese is necessary for antioxidant defence. Manganese, like copper, is needed to make antioxidant enzymes like dismutase and it is also a critical nutrient for sugar metabolism. Food sources are similar to those for copper: nuts and green leafy vegetables.

Gut Advantage

Besides the nutrients, other important elements that benefit the gut are probiotics and prebiotics, as I have said earlier in this book. Good bacteria (probiotic foods or probiotic supplements) and prebiotics (fibre-rich vegetables, grains, psyllium husk and fermented foods) are good foods for the little gut bacteria. Prebiotics should be complemented by the addition of good fats such as virgin coconut oil and desi ghee; they work in synergy to strengthen the gut lining.

Are there foods that increase inflammation? Yes, of course, there are. We need to avoid inflammatory foods, or consume them judiciously. Foods that have an inflammatory effect on the gut are animal proteins, grains such as wheat, rye and corn, processed foods, soy and refined oils. The gut microbiome does not react well to refined sugars either, or chemicals such as preservatives and pesticides.

Detox Foods

In addition, we need foods that detoxify the body and are anti-inflammatory. All the brightly-coloured vegetables, red, purple and green, are rich in antioxidants, which help your body to detox and fight inflammation. Anti-inflammatory foods include good fats, chia seeds and walnuts. Nature has provided us with a wide variety of foods that help our bodies fight off infection and inflammation.

The **kitchen** is indeed the best **pharmacy!** The road to immunity begins from the kitchen.

Natural Remedies

When we were sick or burnt ourselves or got scrapes and bruises, our mothers and grannies usually went straight—into the kitchen! Honey was applied on burns, dahi was used to cool sunburnt skin, isabgol was administered differently for constipation and for diarrhoea, ghee was added to lactating mothers' diets. If you had an upset stomach, they didn't dose you with a number of pills to plug you up; they gave you khichdi and dahi, with aged lemon pickle, or isabgol and dahi, and coconut water to help you hydrate. They knew the digestive value of fermenting foods, pickling vegetables that were in season and of using lemon juice liberally. Homemade pickles and chutneys were the norm.

To fight off viruses (and other invaders), you need to provide the macrophages (defence cells) and soldier cells with energy. Butyrate is the main source of energy for this activity; it helps to rebuild the inside lining of the gut. Butyrate is found in good old traditional fats such as butter and desi ghee. It's not surprising then that grandmas always insisted that you eat plenty of butter and ghee, especially in times of stress, to prevent sickness. Ayurvedic detoxification is also based on fasting followed by the ingestion of ghee to line your gut and fuel your immune cells.

Long before kombucha and sauerkraut became popular as digestives, our home kitchens made tarbooz and kharbooje ki kanji in the summer and kali gajar ki kanji in the winter. There was aam ka panna and phalsa juice to keep the summer heat at bay, and there were chutneys that used mint and coriander with garlic and lemon, and drinks such as haldi-doodh and kadhas that helped keep infections away.

In fact, kadha, a herb and spice-concentrated decoction, is a treasured Indian medicinal secret weapon. Immunity-boosting, it's prepared by slowly simmering together ginger, raw turmeric, tulsi leaves, cinnamon sticks, whole black pepper and cloves. If you are short on time, the concentrate can be kept handy in the refrigerator and a little of it, with warm water, can be drunk regularly.

Flu, as influenza is commonly known, strikes seasonally; it too is caused by a virus and the onset of symptoms is sudden. The similarities with COVID-19 do not end there. The influenza virus also attacks the upper respiratory tract and fever, aches and pains are all common. Of course, we all know now that this novel coronavirus is a more virulent pathogen, and it can cause clotting of the blood, severe respiratory problems and pneumonia.

Considering the current absence of effective therapies for COVID-19, complementary and nutrition therapies assume greater significance to support the body's immune system and prevent complications. Home remedies that help with the flu are also helpful in relieving symptoms. The fact is that newer symptoms are emerging, including skin and gastrointestinal disturbances.

More important, these therapies are very useful prophylactics (preventives) in shoring the body's defences against a major respiratory tract infection from taking hold in the first place. Here's a compendium of some natural food remedies that should find space on every kitchen shelf, and a few traditional and Ayurvedic preparations that help make your immune system stronger:

Amla (Indian gooseberry): This little lime green, sour fruit is the top source of vitamin C; it contains 600 mg per 100 gm, as against about 40 mg per 100 gm in an orange. And the vitamin C in amla is also the most stable; it is preserved even on heating. It's also known to be easily assimilated by the human body.

Aloe Vera: This succulent plant has been known for its benefits; this comes from the seventy-plus vitamins and minerals it contains (several B vitamins, magnesium, zinc, copper, iron and calcium, to name a few). The gel extracted from its leaves has chemicals that help healing because they are anti-inflammatory. They also reduce cholesterol and blood sugars and give the immune system a fillip. These uses do not have major scientific studies to support the use of aloe vera but observationally, many people benefit from the gel. There are some in whom aloe vera can trigger allergies or digestive disturbances.

Giloy: Also known as guduchi, it has gained popularity as a herbal cure for viral fevers. It's propagated in Ayurveda as improving immunity and resistance to infections as well as for its anti-ageing properties.

Hemp Seeds: Hemp belongs to the cannabis family and is often confused with marijuana, though the plant is quite different. Its benefits come from its high protein content (30 per cent) and the fact that its protein is very easily digested. Consumption of its seeds or oil helps fight disease.

Honey: Always known for its medicinal properties, honey is a broad-spectrum antibacterial, antioxidant, anti-inflammatory food. It also has anti-tumour and antiviral properties and helps heal wounds. It's the hydrogen peroxide content and high concentration of natural sugar in honey that gives it antibacterial properties. There is no doubt that it is high in sugar content, but its glycaemic index varies from 32 to 85, depending on the source. Honey loses its efficacy when heated, but can be added to hot drinks.

Manuka Honey: Honey from certain plants, such as the Manuka bush native to New Zealand, is particularly effective in treating digestive disorders. The antibacterial effect of Manuka honey is not from hydrogen peroxide (though it does contain it) but from its high concentration of MGO (a non-peroxide, methylglyoxal). Manuka honey is sold with its UMF (unique Manuka honey factor). A high UMF means higher antibacterial activity because UMF helps the growth of good bacteria. This balance in favour of good bacteria means better gut microbiota and action against the bacteria that cause disease.

Honey can also be used in conjunction with spices to augment its own anti-inflammatory properties. Honey can be used with the following:

Nutmeg—A warming, stimulating and rejuvenating kernel that is grated and added to honey and warm water.

Cloves—These have heating, antifungal and expectorant properties. They are used to make infusions. Had with hot water and honey, the decoctions help relieve symptoms of cold and flu.

Lemon—Lemon juice has antiviral and antibacterial properties and helps stop the progression of infections. Drunk with hot water and honey, it helps soothe sore throats and coughs and colds.

Ginger: Ayurveda is hardly alone in using ginger; other traditional forms of medicine such as Chinese and Unani also use it extensively. Ginger, which contains gingerol and other phenolic compounds, has expectorant and anti-inflammatory properties and is often used to treat sore throats, indigestion and nausea as well as high blood pressure and arthritis. Gingerol helps reduce pain, stimulate circulation and relax blood vessels. It also helps lower cholesterol levels and is anti-clotting. It has the ability to reduce the formation of inflammatory compounds

Tulsi Tea: It's not a surprise that water infused with tulsi leaves is used in Hindu puja ceremonies and that it is added to tea regularly. This herb has many health benefits, among them being that it helps boost the immune system and increase the utilization of oxygen by the cells in the body. It also helps fight off infections—viral, bacterial or fungal—by reducing inflammation. Added to tea, it adds flavour; otherwise, an infusion of just tulsi leaves can be had.

Liquorice (mulethi): The root of this herbaceous plant of the legume family is aromatic and is often used as a flavouring for candied sweets because it is many times sweeter than sugar. Liquorice extract has been used for centuries in traditional medicine to treat indigestion (acidity, constipation and discomfort), coughs, colds and upper respiratory tract irritations. When added to slow-simmered hot infusions, it decreases mucous and coughs. It is also considered useful in treating skin rashes and eczema. Its effects on the body are anti-inflammatory and anti-allergy. But it needs to be consumed in small quantities, so it should be done under the advice of a trained practitioner.

Garlic: Its healing powers have been known for centuries. The knowledge that garlic was good for optimum heart function was known to the first Indian physician, Charak, and the Greek doctor Hippocrates, the father of modern medicine. Scientific studies confirm that garlic contains compounds that lower blood cholesterol and prevent the formation of blood clots that can cause heart attacks. They also help reduce blood pressure.

Turmeric (haldi): Turmeric is a spice Indians know well, used for adding taste and colour to curries and also known for its ability to regulate the immune system. It contains curcumin, which possesses antioxidant, anti-clotting and anti-inflammatory properties. It promotes antiviral and antibacterial activity. This is true Indian yellow gold.

Black Pepper: Black pepper has multiple health-promoting effects, many of which are associated with the relatively high levels of piperine it contains.

Piperine can enhance the oral bioavailability of nutraceuticals in foods. Known to improve healing and stimulate circulation, black pepper releases toxins and reduces congestion. Piperine (also present in white pepper), packs a powerful anti-inflammatory punch. It stimulates circulation and helps in the release of toxins. Honey and black pepper in warm water can help clear congested sinuses. And when turmeric and black pepper, wonderfully effective spices as they are individually, are had together, they give a double boost to the immune system; piperine hugely increases the absorption of curcumin and, thereby, the benefits.

Cinnamon: This spice, made from the inner bark of the *Cinnamomum* tree, has been known for thousands of years to have medicinal properties. Cinnamon helps the immune system and is anti-inflammatory. It stimulates circulation and its ability to improve insulin resistance helps it as an anti-inflammatory and hypoglycaemic agent. These properties make cinnamon especially useful for heart patients and diabetics as well as in boosting immunity.

Black Cumin Seeds (kalonji): These are not actually cumin (jeera) at all, but black caraway or nigella seeds. They too have been shown in studies to significantly lower total and bad cholesterol. The phytosterols present in kalonji seeds strengthen these benefits.

Coriander Seeds (dhania): This spice, regularly used in Indian cooking to add flavour, has also traditionally been used to help lower cholesterol and blood sugar levels. To derive these particular benefits, soak one teaspoon overnight in a small bowl of water and eat them the next morning.

Fenugreek Seeds (methi): An essential ingredient in our traditional spice box, fenugreek seeds have several medicinal properties: they help lower cholesterol and triglyceride levels. They contain saponins that help in regulating blood glucose levels. This spice is also anti-ulcer, antimicrobial and antiparasitic. Methi seeds soaked in water have helped regulate menopause symptoms, protect the liver and promote lactation. And they add taste to food as well. They can be added to pulses and curries, and ground to add to the flour used for rotis.

Cape Gooseberry: Colloquially called 'rasbharries' in India, these little yellow-orange bundles are packed with flavonoids, alkaloids and plant steroids that have strong antimicrobial properties. The rich chlorogenic acid content helps destroy cancer cells. They are also very good sources of vitamin C, A and iron. A power-packed little pop of taste!

Cherries: They are high in iron content and the vitamin C in addition helps the absorption of iron. Highly valued by naturopaths for their natural cleansing properties, they help in flushing out toxins and excess fluid from the kidneys. They are also rich in potassium, magnesium and calcium and low in sodium. They also contain other antioxidants and are high in fibre.

Kokum (Garcinia indica): Used as a sour condiment to flavour south Indian and other Asian curries (preferred over tamarind because of its smoky taste), kokum is an evergreen spice that flourishes in tropical humid conditions. It is also used in beverages and in traditional and Ayurvedic medicines because of its anti-inflammatory, anti-obesity and digestive benefits. It suppresses fatty acid synthesis, inhibits the forming of fat cells and is useful in reducing oxidative stress and insulin resistance—making it anti-inflammatory.

Virgin Coconut Oil (VCO): Coconut oil is actually a protective fat. It's sad that we've stopped stocking it in our kitchens and brought in unhealthy refined fats and hydrogenated margarine instead. I often prescribe VCO to people with immune problems and digestive issues and it has an almost miraculous effect on gut health. It contains lauric acid, which helps the immune system and boosts metabolism.

Desi Ghee: Also a protective fat, desi ghee contains butyrate which, as I have mentioned earlier, is what provides cells that fight infection (macrophages) with the energy to do their job.

Mushrooms, Cordyceps and Shiitake: There are over 1,00,000 species of mushrooms and about 500 of them have been known to the ancients to have medicinal properties. They protect against cardiovascular disease and have antioxidant, anti-inflammatory and antiviral effects.

Japanese studies show that certain mushrooms boost the immune system and help fight infections, cancer and other autoimmune diseases—because of their high content of glutamic acid.

Shiitake is a rich, woody mushroom that is low in calories and rich in minerals such as selenium (portobello and white mushrooms too are rich in selenium) and potassium, zinc, folate and B vitamins. Oyster and shiitake mushrooms are among the best source of beta-glucans. They are commonly used in Asian food and traditional Chinese medicine to boost heart health and increase longevity.

Cordyceps (or caterpillar fungus) is a good source of metabolites—the metabolite cordycepin has high anti-cancer and anti-inflammatory properties. Studies have shown that cordyceps can increase the levels of killer cells (white blood cells that fight viruses and bacteria) significantly. But since natural cordyceps is very expensive, supplements are lab-grown. Mushrooms are a great way to add both flavour and minerals to your food choices.

Apple Cider Vinegar: Fermented apple juice is called cider; further fermentation turns it into apple cider vinegar, an often-used remedy for digestive issues, nasal decongestion, sinus issues and asthma. The malic acid in it is considered to have antiviral and antibacterial properties as well as enzymes that help with digestion. Like lemon juice, though it is acidic in nature, its effect on the body is alkaline, so it improves the pH balance of the body.

Spirulina: A blue-green algae that is considered a superfood; it's rich in protein and vitamins and is a very useful supplement for vegetarians or those on a vegan diet. It has antioxidant properties and can help regulate the body's immune system. It helps promote the growth of healthy gut bacteria in ageing people.

Echinacea: The flower and roots of echinacea have been used by the first nation tribes in Canada and the Europeans to fight infections, the common cold and flu. A typical dose of echinacea is 0.75 to 1.5 ml of tincture per day. However, echinacea can cause some allergies, so it needs to be monitored for reactions.

Gold (swarn) and Silver: Both these precious metals have therapeutic properties. Gold is reputed to increase energy, strengthen the heart muscle and improve memory. It's also used as a nerve tonic. Ayurvedic practitioners use gold to treat anxiety, epilepsy, coronary heart disease, congestive heart failure, arrhythmia and general debility.

Silver (rajata): Silver is an important healing substance due to its cooling and antiseptic properties. According to Ayurveda, it is most useful in treating conditions involving weakness, convalescence or chronic fevers. It is also used to calm inflammatory conditions such as rashes, gastritis, colitis, gut issues and heavy menstrual bleeding.

Traditional Indian Blends

Joshanda: This is a mixture of seven herbs, used in Unani medicine to ease cough, cold and bronchitis. It relieves sore throats and nasal congestion. It is anti-inflammatory and antibacterial.

Chyawanprash: A blend of fifty-one healing ingredients including ghee. A 5000-year-old recipe, chyawanprash is named after Sage Chyawan, who first prepared this formula to impart youth, vigour and longevity. It has anti-stress and anti-ageing properties and is an effective immunity booster and vitalizer. This comprehensive herbal tonic is an amalgam of fifty different herbs and spices (its base is amla, a rich source of vitamin C, which helps bolster immunity; honey acts as a carrier of herbs and helps in their absorption; warming spices such as cardamom, saffron, ginger and cinnamon tonify *agni* or the digestive fire, while liquorice and ghee balance overheating the *pitta dosha*).

Chyawanprash protects the body from respiratory infection by nourishing the mucous membranes and supporting clear respiratory pathways. It also supports the liver in removing toxins from the blood and boosts the production of *ojas*, a subtle essence that is said to be the end product of perfect digestion. It is cooked in a cast-iron skillet, adding iron to the food. The authentic, traditional making of this tonic is key to extracting all the benefits of the herbs and spices. And it can be customized to your specific needs.

Stress, Exercise, Obesity—and Immunity

Stress: Physical or emotional stress can alter hormonal output and immune response. A high level of stress increases the risk of illness and injury in the following year and shortens the life span. Chronic stress also decreases killer cell activity; all these increase the body's susceptibility to disease.

Exercise: Emotional well-being is supported by a proper diet and regular physical exercise. Moderate exercise increases the production of endorphins, the brain's own opiates, which can bolster parts of the immune system and increase killer cell activity. Studies indicate that levels of interleukin-1 and interferon, proteins that send signals for the body to respond to infection or injury, increase after moderate exercise.

However, strenuous aerobic exercise may decrease the efficiency of the immune system and temporarily increase susceptibility to illness by increasing the production of adrenal stress hormones. Among the hormones produced is cortisol, which ordinarily limits inflammation by blocking the immune system. But when there is continued stress, these hormones have elevated levels and the immune system becomes more resistant. The production of protective antibodies (such as secreted IgA, the antibody that protects the intestines and other body cavities against invasion by foreign substances) increases.

Obesity: Former UK Prime Minister Boris Johnson was one of the earliest world leaders to contract COVID-19. Since his recovery, he has been a man on a mission. Johnson is sure his being overweight was a factor in his contracting a more severe form of the infection—and a growing body of evidence backs this up.[5]

A meta-analysis[6] exploring links between obesity and mortality in COVID-19 found that patients with obesity are at a higher risk of mortality from COVID-19 infection. This is not surprising since obesity and comorbidities are a state of inflammation compromising the immune system.

A separate study of people in intensive care units for COVID-19 in the UK found that over 70 per cent were overweight, obese or morbidly obese. A recent analysis of national hospital data in the UK on 1982 COVID-19 patients found that 48 per cent of them were obese. France's chief epidemiologist has said that being overweight is a major risk for people who contract the coronavirus. Therefore, obesity as a factor in exacerbating the severity of COVID-19 is a significant finding. This means that improved eating habits to reduce obesity are essential.[7]

Among other things, the COVID-19 pandemic has brought with it a change in work routines; most people are working from home or in the hybrid model of choosing to work from home or the office. This has resulted in a higher engagement with food, cooking and baking more, and eating more, particularly snacks and sweets. Many of these are high in sugar, fat and carbohydrate content. But if you consume such foods in excess, they can induce insulin resistance and trigger high blood pressure, diabetes, obesity and heart disease. And as obesity has an impact on the severity of COVID-19, a diet rich in such foods can lower your immunity and increase the potential of a more severe infection.

Seven Steps to Success

A checklist of smart habits to build a robust immune system:

1. Plan Your Food Choices

Fruits and Vegetables	Use the rainbow principle: eat brightly-coloured vegetables, green leafy ones as well as root vegetables. A balance of veggies will increase dietary fibre and add disease-fighting phytonutrients to your diet. Eat fruits regularly, but excessive fruit sugar can be counterproductive in some. Avoid fruit juices completely.
Proteins	Prefer plant protein and go easy on animal protein and dairy.
Sprouts and fermented foods	Try and have one of these every day.
Fats	Stick to the good fats, please.

Grains	Avoid inflammatory grains, choose rice, millets, lentils and their flours.
Herbs and spices	Include them judiciously.
Nuts and seeds	Have regularly.
Refined and processed foods	Stay away from them. Consume homemade versions as much as possible.
Sweets	Go easy on sugar in beverages; avoid sweets and desserts, unless it's a celebration. Substitute sugars with dry fruits, honey, or jaggery-based options.

2. **Be Proactive**

   Alkaline Diet: Coronaviruses like the comfort provided by a pH of 6.0 (slightly acidic) in a host body. Research reveals that the coronavirus cannot exist in an alkaline state, even as high as 8.0 (a pH of 7 is considered neutral.) To make the diet alkaline, include plenty of fresh fruits, coconut water and vegetables and avoid excess meat and sugar.[8]

Grow Vegetables: During World War II, there was a massive shortage of vegetables and people converted patches of land into kitchen gardens also called victory gardens. The COVID-19 pandemic is a crisis, but it can also become an opportunity. Take a patch of land from your garden (or use pots on your terrace or balcony) and begin growing vegetables and herbs. Remember that growing your own vegetables makes you eat more vegetables.

3. **Consume Natural Health Foods**
   This is a checklist of useful foods that could be included for regular consumption, but do remember that you are unique. See what works for you.
   Haldi with black pepper in warm water
   Hot lemon water
   Isabgol
   Cow ghee
   Honey
   Chia seeds
   Tulsi
   Giloy
   Neem leaves
   Triphala (if constipated)
   Kadhas

4. **Add Supplements/Vitamins (This is not to be done without consulting a specialist)**
   Supplementation must ensure that optimum levels of vitamins D, C, E, A and B, as well as zinc, are maintained. But considering the toxicity of higher levels of vitamins and minerals, this has to be done

under the supervision of a qualified professional. Nutritional deficiencies, such as anaemia, must be assessed and addressed. Homoeopathy offers excellent, strong and effective immune-building remedies.

5.   **Avoid/Limit/Give Up**
     Beverages: Tea and coffee are beverages that should be taken in limited quantities. They are dehydrating.
     Alcohol: This stimulant may make you feel better, but its intake should be carefully calibrated in today's times. It has a dehydrating effect and too much alcohol consumption lowers immunity levels.
     Smoking: It should be given up at any time, but in a pandemic caused by a pathogen that mainly attacks the lungs and respiratory tract, it poses a serious danger. It compromises the immune system and leaves the lungs wide open to attack.
     Being Inactive: A mainly sedentary lifestyle leads to obesity and lowered immunity. Maintain a regular regime of moderate exercise to get the full benefit.

6.   **Adopt Healthy Habits**
     Try and **synchronize your sleep** and waking patterns with the diurnal rhythm set by nature: sleep early and wake up early.
     Get at least **thirty minutes** of **sunshine** daily to help the body produce vitamin D.
     Get at least **thirty minutes** of **exercise** daily.
     Oil Pulling: This is a traditional Indian technique that has been used for hundreds of years to improve

gut flora naturally. The process is to swish oil around your mouth for fifteen to twenty minutes. Virgin coconut oil or cold-pressed mustard oils are great choices.

Gargle with warm water and salt; **take steam** now and then; **drink warm water** and limit the amount of ice.

Cleanse Your Home Environment: You can keep indoor plants such as aloe vera and mother-in-law's tongue to purify the air inside your home. Camphor, *loban* or other essential aromatic oils can also impart positive energy and a cleansing environment.

Air your rooms regularly.

Create some **humidity** in rooms that are constantly air-conditioned or leave a window open. Also, avoid very low temperatures in air-conditioned rooms; ideally, the temperature should be 23-24 degrees.

7. **Power Up the Mind and Body**
    Practice pranayama and deep breathing. It exercises the diaphragm, improves oxygenation, relaxes the body and activates the pineal gland (which is involved in secreting melatonin, an important anti-inflammatory hormone in the body).
    Meditation: It is a wonderful mental concentrator —a strong, calm mind helps build a strong body.
    Pick any mantra you prefer for your meditation and chanting. Try and keep the same time for your meditation practice; the habit will stand you in good stead.

These seven steps form a critical shield that you can use to protect your body and mind and keep infections at bay. They will help build immunity and resilience, mentally, physically and spiritually.

Last, but not least, remember you are unique and customized advice works best.

HEALTHY RECIPES THAT TICKLE YOUR TASTE BUDS TOO

SALADS

CUCUMBER AND PEANUT SALAD

Ingredients:

2 cucumbers, peeled and finely chopped
3 tbsp peanuts, roasted, peeled and coarsely ground
2 tbsp fresh coconut, scraped
2 tbsp fresh coriander, finely chopped
Juice of ½ lime
1 tsp sugar
Salt as per taste
1 tsp ghee/oil
½ tsp cumin seeds
1 green chilli, cut into big pieces

Method:

Place cucumbers, ground peanuts, fresh coconut and fresh coriander in a mixing bowl. Add salt, sugar and lime juice, and set aside.

Heat ghee/oil in a small pan. Add the cumin seeds and chilli. Take off the heat and swirl the pan to allow the flavours to merge. Add to the salad mix.

Mix well and serve.

BEETROOT SALAD IN A YOGURT DRESSING

Ingredients:

2 medium-sized beetroots
1½ cups thick yogurt/hung curd
1 tsp sugar
Salt as per taste
½ tsp split yellow mustard, coarsely ground
2 tsp fresh coriander, finely chopped

Method:

Scrub the beetroots clean and trim the tops and tails.

Cut into half and cook in a pressure cooker until the pressure has been released twice.

Turn down the heat, release the steam twice and cook for ten minutes. You can also put the beetroots in boiling water until a knife goes through easily, about ten to twelve minutes.

Cool completely. Now, peel off the skin; it should slide off easily.

Chop the beetroot into small cubes and place in a mixing bowl. Add the chopped coriander.

In a separate bowl, whisk the yogurt with the salt, ground mustard and sugar. Combine the yogurt and the beets just before serving.

RAW PAPAYA AND TURMERIC SALAD (SERVES TWO TO THREE)

Ingredients:

1 small raw papaya, peeled and grated
4 tbsp fresh turmeric (haldi), peeled and grated
2 tomatoes, chopped
1 green chilli, chopped fine
1 tbsp raw honey
2 fresh red chillies, chopped fine
Salt as per taste
2 tbsp tamarind (imli) juice
4–5 tulsi leaves
½ cup nuts of any kind—roasted and semi-crushed
1 tsp shatavari powder (an Ayurvedic supplement made from asparagus root)

Method:

Mix the raw papaya, haldi, tomatoes, and green and red chillies in a bowl.

Mix the raw honey with salt and tamarind juice. Add to the salad.

Mix the roasted nuts and shatavari powder. Add to salad and toss well.

Garnish with tulsi leaves.

SAUTÉED BEAN SPROUTS AND TURMERIC SALAD (SERVES SIX)

Ingredients:

½ cup fresh turmeric (haldi), chopped
2 cups bean sprouts
2 tbsp ghee/oil
1 tsp coarsely ground coriander seeds
1 tsp mustard seeds
5–7 curry leaves
Salt
Pepper
Juice of ½ a lemon

Method:

Warm the ghee/oil, add coriander seeds, mustard seeds and any leaves. Stir-fry for a few minutes until the seeds pop.

Add the turmeric and sauté for another few minutes.

Add the bean sprouts and continue to sauté until they soften slightly but don't wait too long or they will wilt.

Add salt and pepper to taste and remove from fire.

Squeeze lemon juice on to the stir-fry before serving.

APPLE AND CELERY SALAD WITH WALNUTS AND MUSTARD VINAIGRETTE

Ingredients:

¼ cup fresh lemon juice
¼ cup fresh mustard paste
4 tsp honey
⅔ cup extra virgin olive oil
1 large bunch celery, with leaves
2 large apples, cut into wedges
¾ cup raw walnuts, chopped
Salt and pepper as per taste

For the Vinaigrette:

In a small bowl, blend the lemon juice, mustard paste and honey.

Gradually whisk in oil.

Season with salt and pepper.

Method:

Trim celery leaves and chop enough to measure one cup.

Thinly slice stalks on deep diagonal.

In a large bowl, combine celery stalks, leaves, apples and walnuts.

Add vinaigrette and toss to coat.

Season with salt and pepper.

SMOOTHIES AND GREEN JUICES

COCONUT SMOOTHIE (SERVES FOUR)

Ingredients:

1 cup purified water
2 cups coconut water
1 grapefruit
1 cup grapes
2 tbsp coconut meat
2 large handfuls of any green leafy vegetable (e.g., mustard, amaranth, methi)
2 large handfuls of lettuce
½ handful arugula

Method:

Start by blending water, coconut water, fruit and coconut.

Add the leafy greens one by one and blend again, until smooth.

Pour the green smoothie into a nut milk bag or cheesecloth.

Gently squeeze it in order to separate the juice from the pulp.

GREEN JUICE I (SERVES TWO)

Ingredients:

2 sweet apples
1 large cucumber

1 small lime
2 handfuls of any green leafy vegetable (or cabbage, chopped broccoli, basella leaves, mustard greens, etc.)
A handful of coriander, with stems
1 tbsp chaat masala/churan or ½ tsp ginger powder

Method:

Put chopped apples, cucumber, lime, greens and coriander into the juicer.

Add chaat masala/ginger powder to the blend.

Pour into a tall glass and enjoy!

GREEN JUICE II (SERVES TWO)

Ingredients:

1 cucumber
½ lemon or lime, chopped
2 stalks of celery
2 stalks spinach/other seasonal green leaves
1 tsp powdered cumin
½–1 inch piece ginger
Extra water

Method:

Chop and add cucumber, lime, celery, spinach, ginger and water to your juicer.

Add cumin powder and blend.

Pour into a tall glass and enjoy!

CITRUS JUICE BLASTER (SERVES TWO)

This refreshing juice blend is perfect for spring-time detox and cleansing. High in fibre, antioxidants and vitamins, it is also the perfect immune booster (diabetics may need to watch the sweetness).

Ingredients:

2 grapefruits
4 oranges
2 lemons
½ tsp red chilli

Method:

Peel the oranges and grapefruits.
Juice them in a juice machine or a citrus press.
Juice the lemon along with the rind if possible.
Mix all ingredients together.
Serve chilled, or at room temperature.

AAM PANNA (MAKES TWELVE GLASSES)

Mangoes are rich in beta-carotene, magnesium and vitamin C, and help in boosting immune function. Kairi panhe or aam panna, a refreshing combination of cooked raw mangoes, jaggery and spices, doesn't just cool you down on a hot day, it also makes an excellent base for cocktails.

Ingredients:

2 medium-sized unripe mangoes (or 1 cup cooked unripe mango pulp)
¾ cup jaggery or raw sugar, grated (use more or less depending on the sourness of the mangoes)
¼ tsp salt
1 large pinch green cardamom powder
1 large pinch saffron strands

Method:

Cook the whole mangoes (with skin) in a pressure cooker with enough water, until soft and mushy.

Peel the mangoes and squeeze out the pulp, discarding the skin and stone.

Place the mango puree and all other ingredients in a blender jar and process until smooth.

Transfer into a sterilized bottle and refrigerate for up to a week.

To serve, put 2 tablespoons of the concentrate in a glass and fill it with cold water and ice.

Add fresh green chilli or mint for an interesting twist.

GREEN SMOOTHIE (MAKES THREE CUPS)

Ingredients:

½ cup water
1 cup pineapple juice
1½ cups (240 gm) green grapes

¼ pear
¼–½ avocado, pitted and peeled
1 floret broccoli
½ cup fresh spinach, washed and cut

Method:

Place all ingredients into a blender.
Blend till smooth and serve in a tall glass.

EVERYTHING SMOOTHIE (MAKES FOUR CUPS)

Ingredients:

½ cup almond/coconut milk
1 cup grapes, red or green
1 medium orange, peeled, halved
½ peach, pitted
½ cup fresh pineapple chunks, core included
½ medium carrot
½ cup fresh broccoli, chopped
½ cup fresh spinach, washed
1 cup frozen unsweetened strawberries
¼ banana, peeled, frozen
1 cup ice cubes

Method:

Place all ingredients into the blender in the order listed and secure the lid.
  Blend till smooth and serve in a tall glass.

KIWI WATERMELON SMOOTHIE (MAKES JUST OVER TWO CUPS)

Ingredients:

1½ cups watermelon, peeled, diced
1 kiwi, peeled, halved
1 date, pitted
1 cup ice cubes

Method:

Place all ingredients into a blender.
Blend for 45 seconds or until smooth.

SHARBATS

AMLA SHARBAT (SERVES THREE OR FOUR)

Ingredients:

1 cup of Indian gooseberry (amla)
½ inch piece ginger
Mint leaves
7 cups water
1 tbsp honey
1½ tbsp roasted cumin powder
1½ tbsp fennel seed powder
1½ tbsp chaat masala (optional)
Black salt, as per taste

Method:

Wash and de-seed the amlas and chop finely.
Wash mint leaves and ginger and chop.
Combine all the ingredients. Blend well.
Serve cold in a tall glass.

INDIAN BAEL KA SHARBAT

Ingredients:

600 gm bael (wood apple) ka phal
1–1½ litres water
1 tsp cumin seed powder
½ tsp black pepper powder
½ cup sugar
½ tsp black salt

Method:

Pound the bael fruit with a pestle, take out the pulp
and discard the hard covering.

Put pulp in a bowl and add ½ litre water.

Soak the pulp for thirty minutes. This makes
it softer.

Mash the pulp with your hands.

Sieve the pulpy juice, pressing so that all the juice is
extracted and only the thick fibres remain.

Add the remaining water.

Add sugar, black pepper, cumin powder and salt.
Mix. Let the sugar dissolve.

Serve chilled.

Tip: If the pulp is too hard, increase the soaking time. It can even be ground but make sure all the seeds are removed or the juice will become bitter.

LIMBU-KESAR SHARBAT (SAFFRON CARDAMOM LEMONADE, MAKES FIFTEEN GLASSES)

On Ranade Road in Dadar, a man would sell lemonade, limbu sharbat, the Marathi version. In the chaos of the street, he would sit quietly on his discoloured plastic stool, confident that the crowds would come to him, the god of sharbat. Even today, when I crave something cool, I think of that lemonade. This is my version: more delicate and with real saffron instead of the street seller's artificial syrup. I keep the concentrate in the refrigerator throughout the summer, ready to be mixed at the smallest excuse of sultry weather.

Ingredients:

1½ cups sugar
2 cups water
1 cup lime juice
½ tsp cardamom powder
12–15 saffron strands

Method:

Dissolve the sugar and water in a pan over a low flame to make a simple syrup, stirring to ensure it does not burn.

Simmer for a few minutes once the sugar is dissolved. The syrup should be only slightly thinner than honey and should coat the back of a spoon lightly.

Add the cardamom and saffron to the syrup and cool completely.

Add the lime juice and stir.

Strain and store in a sterilized bottle in the refrigerator.

To make the lemonade, put three tablespoons of the concentrate in a glass.

Muddle some mint leaves and sprinkle some salt into the glass.

Add ice cubes and fill up with cold water.

Stir and serve immediately.

Also try: Use the same method and proportions to make ginger-lime cordial:

Skip the saffron and cardamom and add bruised, peeled ginger while making the syrup. This syrup has a beautiful blush-pink colour.

KOKUM SHARBAT (KOKUM JUICE CONCENTRATE)

In the Konkan and in some parts of Karnataka, summers mean a bountiful harvest of this beautiful, plum-like cousin of the mangosteen, the kokum (*ratamaba* in Marathi). The syrup is made by simply filling the fruit halves with sugar and is then reduced with a dash of cumin seed powder and salt. This can be stored away for the year. When you come home tired from a trip out in the scorching sun, you simply mix the juice concentrate with cold water and you feel as good as new.

Ingredients:

Kokum fruit
Sugar
Roasted cumin seed powder
Salt as per taste

Method:

Halve the kokum fruit, scoop out the white flesh and discard the seeds.

Fill each half with sugar and pile up the filled kokum halves in a non-metallic jar made of glass or porcelain.

Press down to accommodate as many kokum fruits as you can.

Shut the lid tightly and leave the jar in the sun for a week.

Then strain the liquid out into a thick-bottomed pot.

Season with salt and cumin seed powder and bring to a boil.

Take off the heat, cool completely and fill in sterilized bottles.

Store the bottles in a cool and dark place for several months or refrigerate for up to two years.

To serve, put three tablespoons of kokum syrup in a tall glass and top it with cold water or soda and a few cubes of ice. Stir and serve immediately.

Salt the used kokum skins and leave them to dry in the sun for a few days until completely dry. Use these in curries as a souring agent.

SOL KADHI (KOKUM AND COCONUT MILK DIGESTIVE)

Sol kadhi is that ubiquitous pink beverage served in nearly every fish restaurant along the Konkan coast. The freshly extracted coconut milk, in combination with the tangy, cooling kokum extract, acts as a digestive and palate cleanser.

Ingredients:

½ cup unsweetened kokum extract
3 cups freshly extracted coconut milk (mix of thin and thick)
Salt as per taste
2 cloves garlic
1 small green chilli
1 tsp coriander, finely chopped
2 tsp sugar

Method:

Pound the garlic, chilli and salt to a paste in a mortar with a pestle.

Mix all the ingredients together and adjust seasoning if required.

Serve chilled.

GAJAR KANJI (MAKES EIGHT CUPS)

This traditional north Indian fermented drink is made in the winter with black carrots. As a prebiotic, it is excellent for digestion. If you cannot find black carrots, use regular carrots and add beetroot to give it extra colour.

Ingredients:

5 to 6 medium-sized black carrots or red carrots
2 small beetroots
8 cups water, boiled and strained
1½ tsp red chilli powder
3 tbsp rai/mustard seeds
Black salt

Method:

Rinse and peel the carrots and beetroots and chop into long pieces.

In a glass or ceramic jar, mix all the ingredients.

Cover with a lid and keep the jar in the sun for three to four days.

Stir with a clean wooden spoon every day before turning the jars to the sun.

When the kanji tastes sour, the drink is fermented.

Serve carrot kanji immediately or store in the refrigerator.

SOUPS

BROCCOLI SUNFLOWER SOUP

Ingredients:

4 cups broccoli, chopped
2 cups water
1 tbsp mint (optional)
¼ cup raw shelled sunflower seeds
2 to 3 cloves garlic
2 scallion stalks (spring onions), finely chopped
½ tsp dry oregano
Black pepper, for taste

Method:

Wash and chop the broccoli.

Put the broccoli in a steamer over the water.

Cover and steam until tender and bright green, about five minutes.

While it is steaming, grind the sunflower seeds in the blender into a fine powder. Leave them there.

When the broccoli is done, put it and the cooking water plus the rest of the ingredients in a blender with the ground sunflower seeds and puree.

Heat and serve immediately.

CREAM OF MUSHROOM SOUP WITH GREENS

Ingredients:

1 bunch tender greens, chopped
2 tbsp ghee/oil
¼ tsp black mustard seeds
½ small onion, chopped
1 cup fresh mushrooms, sliced
2 tbsp rice flour/mashed potato
2 cups milk (almond/coconut/rice)
1 tsp sea salt
¼ tsp black pepper

Method:

Wash the greens thoroughly and chop them into one-inch pieces.

Put them in a steamer over boiling water. Cover and steam until tender (five to eight minutes).

While they are steaming, sauté mustard seeds in ghee/oil.

Add chopped onions and sliced mushroom and sauté.

Stir in some boiled and mashed potatoes or rice flour.

Add the cooked greens and the milk and seasoning and simmer for a few more minutes. Serve.

IMMUNITY BOOSTER SOUP

Ingredients:

5 cups water
1-inch fresh ginger root
⅓ cup rice
1 clove
3 whole peppercorns
1 medium carrot, sliced
1 cup raw cabbage or 1 cup fresh greens
1 cup mushrooms
1 pinch cayenne pepper
1 tsp raw honey (optional)

Method:

Bring water to a boil in a saucepan.

Peel and slice the ginger and add to the boiling water, cover and turn heat to low.

Let it simmer while you wash the rice and drain it. Add it to the soup and turn heat up to medium, cover again.

Wash and slice the carrots and mushrooms, and chop the cabbage. Add them to the brew with the clove and peppercorns. Simmer for ten minutes until rice is well-cooked.

Add the cayenne pepper and honey just before serving.

(A special brew during a cold, flu or cough, this soup warms the body and supports the immune system. Cabbage is a rich source of vitamin C and carrot provides generous amounts of beta carotene. Ginger and spices stimulate circulation and digestion.)

FRESH HALDI SOUP

Ingredients:

1 kg tomato, chopped
3 large onions, chopped
2 cloves garlic, chopped
50 gm fresh turmeric
1 tsp sugar
Salt and black pepper, as per taste
Butter as required
200 ml almond milk

Method

Sauté onions and add garlic.
      Cook till light pink, then add chopped tomato.
      Add turmeric, salt, black pepper, butter and sugar.
      Cook in a pressure cooker for two whistles.
      Let it cool and strain.
      Add almond milk. Serve.

SIMPLE ONION SOUP

Ingredients:

2 tbsp ghee
3 large onions, sliced fine
2 cloves garlic, chopped
1 tbsp barley flour
7 cups water
½ bunch fresh parsley, chopped
3 tbsp barley miso
Slices of lemon for garnish

Method:

Put ghee in a large saucepan and add onions and garlic.

Slowly sauté the onions in the ghee over low heat until tender and sweet, about forty-five minutes. Stir occasionally to prevent sticking.

Add flour and stir into ghee (this will be easiest if you clear a space in the centre of the onions so that flour and ghee can be mixed easily without trying to stir the flour into the onions, too).

Gradually add water. Then increase the heat to high and bring the soup to a boil.

Put the miso and about three cups of the soup mixture into a blender.

Add half the chopped parsley and puree.

Stir the blended soup into the rest of the soup, add the rest of the parsley and heat for two minutes. Serve.

SPROUTS AND VEGETABLE SOUP

This popular soup uses beans, but any seasonal vegetables can be added or substituted.

Ingredients:

225 gm green beans
1.2 litres/5 cups lightly salted water
1 garlic clove, roughly chopped
4 almonds, finely chopped
15 gm/⅔ tsp coriander seeds, dry fried
30 ml/2 tbsp vegetable oil
1 onion, finely sliced
400 ml canned coconut milk
2 bay leaves
225 gm bean sprouts (or any other lentil sprouts)
8 thin lemon wedges
30 ml/2 tbsp lemon juice
Salt and ground black pepper

Method:

Cut beans into small-sized pieces.

Bring the salted water to a boil, add the beans and cook for three to four minutes.

Drain, reserving the cooking water. Set the beans aside.

Dry-fry the coriander seeds for about two minutes until the aroma is released.

Finely grind the chopped garlic, almonds and coriander seeds to a paste using a pestle and mortar or in a food processor.

Heat the oil in a wok, and fry the onion until transparent. Remove with a slotted spoon.

Add the nut paste to the wok and fry it for two minutes, without allowing it to brown.

Pour in the reserved vegetable water.

Add the coconut milk, bring to a boil and add the bay leaves. Cook, uncovered, for ten minutes.

Just before serving, reserve a few beans, fried onions and bean sprouts for garnishing and stir the rest into the soup.

Add the lemon wedges, reserved coconut milk, lemon juice and seasoning; stir well.

Pour into individual soup bowls and serve, garnished with reserved beans, onion and bean sprouts.

FOUR-STAR VEGETABLE SOUP

Ingredients:

1 tsp sunflower oil (can use up to 1 tbsp)
½ tsp cumin seeds
⅛ tsp hing (asafoetida)
1½ tsp coriander seeds
2 tbsp dry urad dal
2 cloves garlic, minced (omit for pitta)
1 tsp fresh ginger root, grated
1 carrot, sliced
1 zucchini, sliced

1 cup asparagus/summer squash/string beans/
onions/greens
4 cups water
1 tsp salt or rock salt

Method:

Warm the oil in a medium-sized saucepan.

Add the cumin, hing and coriander seeds and sauté
until brown, for three to five minutes.

Stir in the urad dal, garlic and ginger and sauté for
another two to three minutes.

Add the vegetables and stir.

Pour in the water and bring to a boil. Reduce to
medium heat and cook for half an hour or more. The
longer you cook it, the more tender everything will be.

Add salt and serve.

CAULIFLOWER KADHI

Ingredients:

1 cup cauliflower, diced
3 tbsp rice flour/chana sattu
¼–1 cup onion, chopped
3 cups water
½ tsp fenugreek seeds
1 tbsp ghee or sunflower oil
½ tsp black mustard seeds
2 whole cloves
½ tsp cumin seeds

½ tsp turmeric
4–5 curry leaves, fresh if you can get them
½ tsp fresh ginger root, grated
1 tsp sea salt
1 tsp lime or lemon juice
Fresh coriander leaves, chopped, for garnish

Method:

Put the cauliflower, rice flour/chana sattu, onion and water in a medium kadhai and cook over medium heat until soft, about ten minutes.

Meanwhile, heat the ghee or oil in a small skillet and add the fenugreek, mustard, cloves and cumin.

When the mustard seeds pop, add the turmeric, curry leaves and grated ginger root and cook for an additional thirty seconds.

Add salt and lemon juice to the vegetables in the curry. Cook uncovered for ten to fifteen minutes, stirring occasionally.

Garnish with fresh chopped coriander leaves.

STUFFED TINDA

Ingredients:

500 gm tinda, skin removed, top head removed and make a cross slit at the top
3 tsp fennel seeds
1 tsp sugar
½ tsp turmeric

1 tsp red chilli powder
½ tsp coriander powder
Salt as per taste
½ tsp green chillies
1 tsp ginger, chopped
1 tsp coriander leaves

Ingredients for the masala:

2 tsp desi ghee
1 tsp jeera
1 pinch hing
2 small onions, finely chopped
1 large tomato, chopped
1 tsp ginger, grated
½ tsp red chilli powder
½ tsp coriander powder

Method:

Dry-roast the dry spices and mix. Fill into the slits on the tinda.

Heat ghee in a pressure cooker.

Fry onions till golden, add tomato and ginger.

Add sugar, salt, green chillies, chilli powder and coriander powder and cook till a gravy is formed.

Add tinda at the end and cook for one or two whistles.

Garnish with fresh coriander and serve.

KOKUM CURRY

Ingredients:

10 to 12 kokum fruit
2 cups water
2 cups coconut milk
Salt
½ tsp mustard seeds
1 tsp cumin
12 sprigs curry leaves
1 pinch asafoetida (hing)
4 to 5 garlic cloves, slightly crushed
2 Kashmiri red chillies
2 tbsp ghee/oil
Coriander leaves for garnish

Method:

Soak the kokum in half a cup of water for thirty minutes.

Then crush and squeeze them completely to get a pinkish-red extract.

Add two cups of water and coconut milk to the kokum extract.

Add salt and stir.

Heat ghee/oil.

Add mustard seeds and cook till they splutter.

Add cumin and let it sizzle.

Add the garlic, asafoetida, red chillies and curry leaves.

Pour this tempering over the kokum coconut milk mixture and then garnish with coriander leaves.

Serve with boiled rice/millets and vegetables.

FENUGREEK AND RADISH CURRY

This is a great late-winter veggie dish. Besan and garlic give it a unique flavour

Ingredients:

1 bunch fresh fenugreek (methi) leaves
7 to 8 red radishes, chopped into quarters
2 cloves garlic, chopped
1 tbsp besan flour
Salt as per taste
1 pinch jaggery
½ tsp turmeric
½ tsp cumin
1 tsp ghee/mustard oil
1 tomato, chopped (optional)

Method:

Heat the oil in a pan and add cumin until it sizzles.

Add garlic cloves, radish and a little water to cook the radishes halfway through.

Add the besan and stir until it is a little golden-brown.

Add the methi leaves and seasonings.

Simmer on low heat, but be careful not to burn it.

Add a little water if it seems too dry.

Add tomatoes for more depth of flavour.

Serve warm with rice/millets.

ROTIS

RAGI ROTI

Also called finger millet or nachani, this is a high-nutrient iron and calcium grain, native to south India. It's an excellent alternative for those who are intolerant to wheat.

Ingredients:

½ cup of ragi (nachani or finger millet) flour
3 tbsp spring onions, finely chopped (green and white parts)
¼ cup carrot, grated
1½ tsp yogurt (dahi)
½ tbsp green chilli paste
Salt

Method:

In a bowl, combine all the ingredients with water and knead into a smooth dough.

Divide the dough into four equal portions.

Roll each portion out into a roti.

Place the roti on a non-stick pan and turn over in a few seconds.

Cook the other side for a few more seconds.

Lift the roti with a pair of flat tongs and roast over an open flame until brown spots appear on both sides.

Repeat with the remaining portions to make more rotis.

Serve hot.

BHAKRI (SORGHUM FLATBREAD)

Ingredients:

2 cups jowar (sorghum) flour
1 cup hot water (can adjust according to flour)
Salt as per taste

Method:

Place flour in a large mixing bowl and make a well in the centre.

Add salt.

Add hot water slowly in small batches and knead into a soft dough.

Make small walnut-sized balls and keep them covered.

Roll out each ball on a floured surface. You could also roll it in between sheets of butter paper or flatten it with water on your palms.

Slide it out on to a tawa. Sprinkle the top with water immediately to prevent cracking.

Flip after five seconds. Cook till light brown spots appear.

Remove from tawa and cook on flame till it puffs up.

Remove and serve hot brushed with ghee or butter.

(Useful tip: Use freshly ground flour. If the flour is too old, the bhakri will crack and taste bitter. Also, use boiling hot water; this helps the dough cook a little and it has more strength.)

Another kind of bhakri that is popular in the Khandesh region is the kalnyaachi bhakri, which is made of a flour mix containing split black lentils (urad dal) along with bajra (pearl millet) and/or jowar. The stickiness from the split black lentils makes the bhakri easy to pat.

KHICHDI (HEALTHY INDIAN GRAIN AND PULSE STEW)

Khichdi is integral to Ayurvedic nutritional healing. These are relatively simple stews of rice and/or millet with dals, which are suitable for almost everyone. There are endless variations depending on the herbs, spices and vegetables used. In the Ayurvedic cleansing therapy of Panchakarma, they are eaten with ghee because of their ease of digestion and assimilation. Almost all diets for convalescence contain khichdi. It's best eaten freshly cooked. It has been conferred 'National Dish' status.

Ingredients:

Accompaniment, lubrication and assimilation: Ghee

Spices that enhance digestibility and boost immunity:
Asafoetida (hing): aids assimilation, potent carminative
Bay leaf: digestive
Black mustard seeds: digestive, anti-inflammatory
Black peppercorns: digestive, carminative
Cardamom: calms and stimulates digestion
Cinnamon: digestive, anti-inflammatory
Cloves: digestive, anti-inflammatory

Coriander: soothing, carminative, digestive
Cumin: carminative, digestive
Fennel: digestive, cooling and tonifying to the stomach
Fenugreek: digestive, anti-inflammatory
Garlic: strengthening, anti-infective, anti-clotting
Ginger: potent digestive stimulant, anti-inflammatory
Curry leaves: cooling, clear and remove wastes (detoxifying)
Saffron: digestive, immunity booster
Turmeric: anti-infective, anti-inflammatory

Several of these can be combined with split moong dal, rice and vegetables. Other lentils and grains can be used. Cook until both lentil and grain are very soft but not gummy. Allow your intuition, creativity and self-knowledge to guide you in the combinations

BASIC WARMING KHICHDI

Ingredients:

½ cup basmati rice
¼ cup split moong dal
6 cups water
1 tbsp desi ghee/virgin coconut oil/extra virgin olive oil
1 tsp cumin seeds
1 pinch hing
1 tsp coriander seeds
¾ tsp cardamom seeds

1 tsp black peppercorns
1 bay leaf
2 more tbsp ghee
1 small stick cinnamon
¼ tsp ground cloves
1 tsp salt, rock salt if you can get it
1 tbsp fresh ginger root, grated
½ small onion, chopped
1–2 cloves garlic (optional)
½ tsp ground cumin
2–4 cups fresh vegetables: carrots, greens, string
beans or zucchini are possibilities, diced fine
2 more cups water, as needed

Method:

While this is an imposing list of ingredients, it's actually
easy to make.

Wash the rice and split moong dal until the rinse
water is clear.

Warm a tbsp of ghee in a medium saucepan and
add the cumin seeds and hing. Lightly brown them.

Add the rice, moong and water and bring to a boil.
Cook for about forty-five minutes.

Warm the two tablespoons of ghee in a small skillet.

Add the coriander, cardamom, peppercorns and
bay leaf and sauté for two to three minutes.

Then stir in the rest of the spices and the onion
(and garlic, if you use it).

Put the sautéed spices in a blender with a little (½ cup or less) water and grind well.

Pour this spice mixture into the rice and dal mix.

Rinse out the blender with the last two cups of water and add it to the khichdi as well.

Add the vegetables. Cook for twenty minutes or more.

IMMUNITY KHICHDI

Follow the recipe for Basic Warming Khichdi with the following changes:

Wash two medium sweet potatoes and dice into ½ to 1-inch pieces.

Add ½ teaspoon ajwain (carom seeds) and sauté with the cumin and hing.

Add the sweet potato when you add moong, rice and water. Again, cook for about forty-five minutes.

Omit the bay leaf and fresh ginger and cut the cardamom to ¼ teaspoon (1 pod).

Cut the ghee or oil in the second step to 1 tbsp and add the coriander, cardamom, peppercorns and ¼ tsp dry ginger. Sauté for two to three minutes.

Then stir in the rest of the spices, onion and four cloves of garlic.

Follow the rest of the recipe as described.

If you like, you can add one tablespoon of flaxseeds or chia seeds in the last fifteen minutes of cooking to enhance clearing of the lungs.

This is an excellent immunity-boosting dish for fighting flu and phlegm. Ajwain and ginger work to decongest the lungs, while the onion and garlic warm and stimulate the immune system and circulation. Sweet potato is rich in beta-carotene, which supports the immune system.

THERAPEUTIC KHICHDI

Ingredients:

½ cup dry chickpeas (white chana)
6 cups water
1 pinch hing
1–2 tbsp ghee
½ tsp black mustard seeds
1 tsp cumin seeds
1 tsp turmeric
1 large onion, chopped
2 cloves garlic, minced
1 cup rice/millets
2 to 4 more cups of water (as needed)
1 turnip, chopped (optional)
1 carrot, chopped
1 cup cabbage or broccoli, chopped
¾ tsp sea salt
1 tsp ground coriander
1 tbsp sesame seeds

Method:

Wash the chickpeas and rice.

Put the chickpeas, water and hing in a pressure cooker and bring to pressure. Cook for thirty minutes on medium heat.

Meanwhile, warm the ghee in a medium-sized skillet and add the mustard and cumin seeds.

When the mustard seeds pop, add the turmeric, onion and garlic. Stir over low heat for two to three minutes. Add the rice and stir. Set aside.

When the chickpeas are cooked, open the pressure cooker and add the spiced rice mixture.

Add the turnip and extra water. Cook for forty-five minutes or until the rice is tender.

Add the rest of the vegetables and spices and simmer for another fifteen minutes.

Chickpeas calm irritated or inflamed lungs; carrot, cabbage and broccoli add vitamins A and C.

DIGESTIVE KHICHDI

Ingredients:

½ tsp cumin seeds
2 tbsp ghee or sunflower oil
3 bay leaves
1 tsp turmeric
1 tsp coriander seeds
1 tsp oregano, dry
½ tsp sea salt
1 stick kombu (optional). Kombu is a seaweed that helps in detoxifying heavy metals
1 tsp fresh ginger root, grated

½ cup basmati rice
¼ cup split moong dal
4–6 cups water
2 cups fresh vegetables, such as carrots, zucchini or summer squash, diced

Method:

Wash the rice and dal until the water is clear.

Warm the ghee in a medium saucepan.

Add the cumin seeds, bay leaves, coriander and oregano. Brown slightly, until aromatic (you can smell them).

Stir in turmeric, rice and dal. Add water, salt, kombu (if used) and ginger. Simmer covered over medium heat until dal and rice are soft, about 1 hour.

Add vegetables and cook until tender, for fifteen to twenty minutes.

Garnish generously with fresh chopped coriander leaves. A little ghee can be added after cooking

COCONUT CHIPS

Coconut chips are a perfect low-carb snack that can be had at any time.

Ingredients:

1 fresh coconut

Method:

Preheat the oven to 160°C/325°F.

Drain the coconut juice, either by piercing one of the coconut eyes with a sharp instrument or by breaking it carefully.

Slice the flesh into wafer-thin shavings, using a food processor, mandoline or sharp knife.

Sprinkle these evenly all over one or two baking sheets and sprinkle with salt. Bake for about twenty-five to thirty minutes or until crisp, turning them from time to time.

You may try baking sliced beetroot/parsnips/sweet potatoes in the same way (air fryers are also a good way to cook such chips).

Cook's tip: This is the kind of recipe where the slicing blade on a food processor comes into its own. It is worth preparing two or three coconuts at a time and freezing the surplus chips. These can be cooked from frozen but will need to be spread out well on the baking sheets before being salted. Allow a little longer for frozen chips to cook.

HOT AND SWEET CASHEW NUTS

Ingredients:

1 tbsp groundnut oil
2 tbsp clear honey
250 gm cashew nuts
⅓ cup desiccated (dry) unsweetened coconut

2 small fresh red chillies, seeded and finely chopped
Salt and ground black pepper

Method:

Heat oil in a wok or kadhai. Stir in the honey.

After a few seconds, add the cashews and coconut and stir-fry until both are golden brown.

Add the chillies with salt and pepper to taste.

Toss until all the ingredients are well mixed.

Serve warm or cooled in paper cones or saucers.

Variations: Almonds also work well or choose peanuts for a more economical snack.

BOILED PEANUTS WITH CUMIN AND COCONUT

Ingredients:

2 cups peanuts/chana/mixed seeds
2 tsp oil
2–3 green chillies, diced
1 tsp cumin seeds
½ tsp roasted cumin seed powder
Salt as per taste
1 tsp sugar
2 tbsp fresh coconut, grated
2 tbsp fresh coriander, finely chopped

Method:

Cook the peanuts in a cup of water with a good pinch of salt in a pressure cooker until the pressure has been released twice.

Then, turn down the flame and cook for another five minutes. Allow the pressure to release naturally. The peanuts should be fully cooked but not too soft.

Heat the oil in a pan.

Add the cumin seeds and green chillies. Sauté for two to three minutes and add the boiled peanuts and then the roasted cumin seed powder. Adjust seasoning to your taste.

If the peanuts appear too dry, add half a cup of water. Cover and cook for five to eight minutes until the peanuts are soft.

Add sugar, coconut and coriander and toss. Serve hot.

CARROT AND COCONUT CHUTNEY

Ingredients:

1 cup carrot, grated
¼ cup coconut, grated
½ to ¾ cup fresh turmeric, grated
1½ tbsp urad dal
5–6 red chillies
1 small tamarind
1 tbsp mustard oil
Salt
Coriander leaves, chopped for garnish

Method:

In a pan, heat oil and fry the urad dal and red chillies until they turn golden brown.

Add the turmeric and grated carrots. Sauté until the raw smell disappears.

Transfer the sautéed items into a food processor or mixer and grind with coconut, tamarind, salt and water into a smooth chutney.

Top with chopped coriander.

POHA CUTLETS (MAKES TEN PIECES)

Ingredients:

1 cup thick poha

1 large potato or ¾ cup mashed potatoes

1 small carrot, finely chopped or grated or ¼ cup finely chopped or grated carrots

4–5 blanched French beans, finely chopped or ¼ cup steamed or boiled green peas

1 small onion finely chopped or ¼ cup finely chopped onion

1 tbsp chopped coriander leaves

½ tsp ginger–garlic paste

¼ tsp turmeric powder

¼ tsp red chilli powder

¼–½ tsp garam masala powder

½ tsp dry mango powder (amchur)

1 tsp white sesame seeds

1 pinch sugar (optional)

3 tbsp oil for pan-frying
Salt as per taste

Method:

Take thick poha and rinse it once or twice.

Soak the poha in water just about covering it for three to four minutes.

Using a strainer, drain all the water from the poha.

The poha should get softened well but there should be no water in it. Use a strainer to drain all the water.

Poha Cutlet Mixture:

Steam or boil potato in a pressure cooker or steamer till it is softened and cooked really well. Peel it when still warm.

Mash well with a fork or with your hands.

Add the finely chopped vegetables—carrots, blanched French beans, onion, coriander leaves and ginger-garlic paste.

French beans need to be blanched before you add them to the cutlets.

Add the poha.

Now add turmeric powder, red chilli powder, garam masala powder, dry mango powder, white sesame seeds, a pinch of sugar (optional) and salt as per taste.

Mix everything well. Check the taste and add more salt or spices if required.

Shape into small cutlets. Pan-fry cutlets from both sides for a few minutes.

HUMMUS

Ingredients:

2 cups boiled chickpeas, drained
¼ cup (35 gm) raw sesame seeds
1 tbsp olive oil
¼ cup (60 ml) lemon juice
3 garlic cloves, peeled
1 tsp cumin
Salt

Method:

Place all ingredients except salt, into a blender.
    Grind to a smooth paste and season with salt.
    Serve garnished with a drizzle of olive oil.
    Accompany with crackers, bread, falafel or vegetable sticks.

PESTO (BASIL PASTE)

Ingredients:

½ cup (120 ml) olive oil
½ cup (50 gm) grated Parmesan cheese
3 medium garlic cloves, peeled
2 cups fresh basil leaves
3 tbsp pine nuts/any nuts
Salt and pepper as per taste

Method:

Place all ingredients in a blender and blend till it's a fine paste.

Use with vegetables/rice/pasta.

AMLA CHUTNEY

Ingredients:

½ kg amla
1 tsp cardamom
1 tsp freshly ground black pepper
¼ cup finely chopped almonds

Method:

Wash amla and cook in a pressure cooker with the spices, until two whistles have sounded.

Remove seeds and mash.

Add almonds and cool.

Store in a jar in the refrigerator and take a spoonful in the morning with 1 tsp honey.

JAMUN CHUTNEY

Ingredients:

1 small bowl jamun pulp
4 cloves garlic
1 tsp ginger, chopped
1 tbsp green chillies, chopped

1 tbsp peanuts without skin
½ tsp white salt
½ tsp rock salt
A few drops of honey
½ tsp roasted fenugreek seeds
½ tsp cumin seeds
½ tsp lemon juice
½ tsp oil
5–8 curry leaves

Method:

Mix all the ingredients, except oil, cumin seeds and curry leaves.

Put into a blender and make a fine paste. Put into a serving bowl.

Heat oil and add cumin seeds and curry leaves. Pour over the chutney. You can also add some roasted sesame seeds as a garnish.

RICE CHUTNEY

Ingredients:

Rice (congee variety)
For tempering: desi ghee, hing, cumin, ajwain and salt

Method:

Drain the starch water from boiled rice and leave it overnight to ferment.

Cook for five to ten minutes and temper with desi ghee, hing, cumin, ajwain and salt.

ALMOND POPPY PASTE

Ingredients:

1 cup soaked and peeled almonds
5 tsp poppy seeds, soaked for eight hours
2 tsp crushed or powdered cardamom
10–12 crushed black peppercorns

Method:

Combine all the ingredients and grind in a blender with minimum water to make a fine paste.

Store in a refrigerator and take 1 teaspoon daily.

PAUSHTIK LADDOO (PEANUT AND JAGGERY LADDOOS)

Method:

Combine ground peanuts with grated jaggery and knead the mixture until it binds well into a soft dough.

Grease your palms with a little oil/ghee and shape into balls.

Eat immediately or store for two to three days in an airtight box in a cool and dry place. Great for kids and the elderly.

NACHNI AND DATE LADDOOS

These are an excellent high-nutrient fix for the sweet tooth. Rich in calcium and iron, they are best had in the daylight hours as an afternoon snack.

Ingredients:

1 cup millet flour (ragi/nachani)
1 cup dates, seeded and finely chopped
2 tsp poppy or sesame seeds
¼ tsp ground cardamom
5 tbsp ghee

Method:

Heat three tablespoons of ghee in a pan over medium heat.

Add the millet flour and cook, stirring continuously until the flour turns golden brown.

Remove from heat and transfer to a mixing bowl.

Dry-roast the poppy or sesame seeds in the same pan and then add to the mixing bowl.

Heat the remaining two tablespoons of ghee over medium heat, add the dates, sauté for two minutes and transfer to the mixing bowl.

Add ground cardamom and knead together. While still warm, divide it up. Grease your palms and shape into round laddoos.

Chapter XIII

Casebook of the Diet Detective

Much of what I do in my practice is investigate. In this journey of detection, serology (blood tests) and other scans have a role to play, as they are useful in giving us the levels of various markers. But most important is getting the patient to describe all their symptoms exhaustively and finding the dietary clues that might be triggering internal trouble. This means asking questions, a lot of them. And sifting through everything, to separate the vital pieces of information.

So, often, I find myself feeling like a diet detective; satisfaction comes from being able to solve the case and find the dietary criminal lurking inside. It could be inflammation caused by a food intolerance, inflammation because of insulin resistance or a deficiency caused by malabsorption (leaky gut). Very often, a combination of these.

From my practice's case book, I have selected a number of varied instances, which illustrate how an extremely wide array of symptoms and rather diverse disorders and diseases were linked to the functioning of the gut (in conjunction with the other three G-forces). Some cases needed a deep dive into testing to find the culprits; in some histories, detailed Q and As sufficed for the detective to solve the crime; in a few, financial considerations did not allow for expensive testing, so a simpler approach of elimination of certain foods and observation of symptoms was adopted.

What was deeply satisfying, however, was the kind of health transformation that was realized through the combination of identification, elimination, supplementation and dietary planning. In addition, mostly, the other lifestyle factors have remained constant, such as exercise, sleep, stress, pesticides in food, pollution and disease.

The gratification comes at many levels. In all the cases, one can understand the origin of the problem. From there on, joining the dots is easy.

The improvement/removal of symptoms is accompanied by a reduction in the pill burden or complete removal of pills. In all instances, people are eating less than before, and they report feeling more energetic and positive about their health.

Interestingly, whenever there is re-exposure to inflammatory foods, the symptoms reappear. They then report increased appetite, sugar cravings, bloating, lower levels of energy and mood swings. The weight goes up; sugar levels become more unstable in diabetics; in those with digestive issues, symptoms recur and the skin flares up—depending on the severity of the exposure. It usually takes a week to ten days for things to settle down again.

The Case of the Perimenopausal Educationist

Mrs J., five feet five inches tall, had been an active and productive hill woman, used to walking over five km a day, with nary an ounce of extra weight. But she had trouble conceiving and after she had a baby (at thirty-five), she developed a weight problem.

Presenting Symptoms

- At forty-five, perimenopausal, developed endometrial hyperplasia and anxiety and was put on hormone therapy and antidepressants
- Bloating, fatigue, poor appetite and thirst (ate only 1500 calories) but was 76 kg
- Anxiety, prone to psychosomatic disorders, episodic borderline high blood pressure

She was vegetarian; we applied grain science, eliminating wheat and cross-sensitive cereals and suggested alternatives, and added supplementary nutrients. She soon achieved a return of her energy levels and lost 5 kg in three months. Her blood pressure levels normalized and the anxiety resolved.

The Case of the Pained Back

Mr G., forty-six, was referred to us by his physiotherapy clinic because he could find no relief for the pain in his lower back. At five feet nine, he weighed 96 kg and had a BMI of 30, marking him as obese.

Presenting Symptoms

Inflammation in the sacroiliac joint in the lower back and such severe pain that he could not exercise at all.

Bloodwork showed thyroid antibodies were positive with high PTH (parathyroid hormone) levels. Iron and vitamin D3 levels were low, eosinophils and uric acid were high and intestinal inflammation marker faecal calprotectin was 67 (it should be under 50). He also had abnormal cholesterol levels.

All these markers indicated inflammation. We eliminated inflammatory grains completely from his diet and soon, all the parameters that were high either came within normal range or close to it. He lost 7 kg over four months and his aches and pains resolved. He got his normal life back.

The 'Sendha Namak' Case

Mrs M., a forty-four-year-old architect, consulted the clinic for a range of issues. She was not obese (BMI was 24) and her diet was conventionally balanced, low-cal and low-carb.

Presenting Symptoms

- Vitiligo (for nine years)
- Low-grade fever, water retention, with swelling on face, hands and feet

- Had irregular periods; bloating and gas in the last year and recent acne
- Sometimes she would just choke
- The key clue: as long as she consumed sendha namak (rock salt), she was fine. But if she ate regular salt, her hands, face and body would swell up. She was so sure about the association that she carried her own salt everywhere.

To the diet detective, this was the key clue that helped solve her case. It revealed she had a severe magnesium deficiency (rock salt contains many minerals, including magnesium). Her bloodwork showed as much, plus very low vitamin D and critically low vitamin B12 levels. Her CRP and pancreatic enzyme lipase were slightly elevated, which indicated inflammation.

Clearly, gluten sensitivity and a leaky gut had created this deficiency. The elimination of inflammatory grains and the addition of magnesium supplements immediately began reducing the swelling; her fever and bloodwork became normal. More important, her skin began to re-pigment itself, reducing the vitiligo patches. Since going gluten-free was so essential for her, her mother did the same to emotionally support her. Her improvement was so life-changing that she began giving talks about it in industry fora.

The Case of the 'Otherwise Thin' Lady

Mrs G., just over forty, was tall at five feet eight. But she had an exceptionally large belly, a BMI of 28.5 and weighed 86 kg.

Presenting Symptoms

- Low appetite, a low-cal diet but unable to lose weight
- Poor immunity (had frequent urinary infections) and severe knee pain that wasn't resolved by physiotherapy
- A history of severe hair fall, food allergies and PCOS

Investigation revealed very low vitamin D and B12 levels, borderline thyroid function and dyslipidemia (her LDL, which is the bad cholesterol level, was high and HDL, the good cholesterol, was as low as 33). We resolved her problem by removing inflammatory grains and replaced nutrients by adding vitamin and mineral supplements. Her weight came down to 65 kg and her waist from over 39 inches to 32.5. Her HDL levels rose, her energy levels soon improved, the knee pain resolved and she began exercising regularly.

But she came back after a trip to South Korea and rushed to meet me, wearing chappals in the dead of winter; her feet were so swollen she couldn't get into a pair of shoes. And her knee pain was back. I asked her what she had been eating. The culprit? Soya in tofu and soy sauce (which contains gluten and soy). Within a week of returning to her regular dietary pattern, the swelling vanished and the pain disappeared. She's far more careful now when she travels.

The Case of the Prodigal Patient

Mrs K., fifty-five, a former patient, returned to consult us after a decade's gap—this time, with a warrant for bariatric surgery. She had a bad case history: she had lost some weight in her earlier innings but then stopped coming. She relapsed on the diet front, regained the lost weight and more (reached 120 kg), and then was put on insulin (and the dosage had spiralled higher and higher).

Presenting Symptoms

- Morbid obesity
- Diabetes was so severe that insulin had increased to 100 units a day
- Kidney disease
- Her physician had told her bariatric surgery was her only option

I told her that we could remove the offending gluten-containing grains and foods but that at her current insulin doses, her blood sugar would plummet and she could collapse. But her physician absolutely refused to reduce the prescribed amounts. Eventually, she took the call herself and reduced her insulin. Within three months of dietary change, she lost 10 kg and was down from taking 100 units—to **NIL**. Her diabetes had been reversed as well as the kidney malfunctioning. Over the course of a year, she lost a grand total of 35 kg. Of course, the bariatric surgery was not needed!

A Case of PCOD

Ms S., thirty-nine, had been diagnosed with PCOD two years before she consulted me. She was on medication for the condition. When she came in 2018, her weight was 63 kg, she stood at five feet three and her BMI was 23. She was not obese, but her waist measurement was 35.5 inches, which was higher than normal.

Presenting Symptoms

- PCOD: her cysts were not improving, despite medication and her periods were very irregular
- Had a thyroid nodule
- Severe acidity; was on antacids

Blood tests showed low haemoglobin (9.3) and abnormal cholesterol levels. We changed her to a no-gluten, low-dairy diet. She was vegetarian, so we did not remove dairy products altogether but encouraged her not to have them. In less than a month, she reported feeling much better and had a normal period. When she went for a scan, her cysts had disappeared, as had her thyroid nodule. Her haemoglobin went up to 12.7, with just homoeopathic iron added. Soon, she also lost some weight and her waist came down to 32.5 inches.

The interesting thing about her case was that by elimination of inflammatory grains and supplementation, it wasn't just her symptoms that had resolved but the actual cysts had vanished, as seen on a sonography. Since then, she has followed the modified grain diet, staying gluten-free and dairy free. She continues to follow up with us.

What was even more gratifying was that when she visited her physician for a routine check-up, he tried to locate her thyroid nodule and this too had vanished—to the utter surprise of the doctor!

A Case of Chronic Constipation

A 10-year-old girl came in with severe constipation; she would strain so much that she would get blood in the stool. She'd been taken to paediatricians and gastro specialists and been prescribed laxatives and a high-fibre diet. But nothing worked and she began to get a protruding belly. By the time she came to us, she was obese. As a child, she had been breastfed, but she was so underweight that at six months, she had been given a special syrup to help her gain weight, after which she gained weight steadily (she then gained 20 kg).

Presenting Symptoms

- Chronic constipation
- Low immunity
- History of hair fall and severe itching on the body

Blood tests revealed low vitamin D3, critically low magnesium (when bloodwork shows low levels, it means the tissues are starved of the mineral) and her anti-gliadin antibody test (for wheat intolerance) was positive. We eliminated the gluten and gave her a normal diet with modified grains and vegetables, and supplemented with magnesium. By the next follow-up (in two weeks), her stools were already becoming soft and regular. And by the second visit (in a month), her other issues of itching and hair fall were also resolving and the constipation was a thing of the past. Her mother was eternally grateful for this resolution to her child's daily suffering.

A Case of Diabetes Control

A fifty-six-year-old gentleman, Mr H., had diabetes since he was thirty-five. He was on forty units of insulin daily. Not obese, he did have a fatty liver and was carrying extra belly fat (girth was 35.5 inches).

Presenting Symptoms

- Diabetes for twenty years
- History of sinusitis, low immunity
- Dry skin and mild constipation

Bloodwork showed the glycosylated Hb (HbA1C) was 7.2, despite the insulin shots he had been taking for several years. His cholesterol levels were abnormal and his haemoglobin was low. We put him on a modified grain diet and cut out the dairy as well. In just six weeks, the sugar levels were better controlled and the need for insulin came down to—ZERO. And even without the insulin, on his next blood test, after eight weeks on the changed diet, the HbA1C was 6.8.

For the last two years, he's been off insulin; his diabetes is controlled by dietary change alone. He is now a happy man, insulin-free and his diabetes is under control.

The Dramatic Case of the Man with Vitiligo

Mr V., thirty-six, came in four years ago. He was really obese, at 109 kg (height was five feet nine). His BMI was 35 kg/m2 and waist measurement came in at over 47 inches. He came for weight loss but clearly had other health issues. He had abnormal liver function tests (SGPT, SGOT and VGTP were all elevated) and had low vitamin D and vitamin B12. Ferritin levels were too high (a sign of inflammation). Uric acid too was on the high side.

Presenting Symptoms

Most significantly, he was all 'white', or de-pigmented, a condition called vitiligo or leucoderma, since he was eight years old.

When we tested him for wheat sensitivity, his celiac marker was negative but the anti-gliadin antibody was positive (this indicated a non-celiac wheat sensitivity or NCWS). He lost weight, though quite slowly.

But the dramatic change was elsewhere. The wheat sensitivity results take time, but even without them, when he first came in, I put him on a low carbohydrate diet because both his parents were diabetic. We gave him a low glycaemic index flour which, by default, did not contain wheat. By the time of his third check-up, he was getting brown spots on his arms. In four months, he had full brown patches on his face and was re-pigmenting rapidly. I mentioned to him my observation about wheat leading to his vitiligo and that it does have a genetic basis. He then informed me that his son, at age four, was also showing the same skin issue.

But his face was looking patchy and spotty, and his wife did not like this. He went back to eating wheat and the pigmentation soon vanished. His dermatologist dismissed the diet connection, so he stopped coming.

The Case of the Autistic Child

A nine-year-old boy came in, having been diagnosed with autism and ADHD. He was already on medication for the disorders, prescribed by his physician (a paediatric psychiatrist). Autistic kids often harm themselves; this boy would bang his head against a wall for hours, twice a day at least. He had bleeding wounds on the head from the injuries.

Presenting Symptoms

Uncontrollable stomach ache and nausea, as well as the head-banging.

His celiac markers were negative. The anti-gliadin antibody test was positive (NCWS) and the food intolerance test also showed milk intolerance. Dairy was removed from his diet and grains modified to eliminate inflammatory ones, such as wheat and cross-sensitive grains. Gut-building foods, including virgin coconut oil and vitamin and mineral supplements, were added. Within a week, the head-banging reduced to half the duration. In a few weeks, it stopped. The connection between diet and symptoms was so obvious that when he ate a regular chocolate muffin given inadvertently by a teacher in school, there was a resurgence of the behaviour, which then took months to resolve.

We have been following up with him now for over three years; his issues are generally resolved. We keep him on a no-sugar, no-dairy and gluten-free grain diet. He's getting supportive therapy, but much less. Even his doctor has been focusing on gut health to keep him fully functional in all respects.

A Case of Ulcerative Colitis

Mr C. came to us in 2016; he'd been on medication for ulcerative colitis for six years. He was also taking multivitamins, calcium and iron supplements and a protein powder. His BMI was 25. Investigation showed elevated CRP (12.3) and Hb was 12.7, on the low end of normal.

Presenting Symptoms

- Colitis with continuous bleeding, despite years of medication

- Passing stools many times a day
- Weight loss

His celiac markers were negative. When we started the elimination of inflammatory grains and dairy, and the rebuilding diet, the frequency of motions began decreasing. He began to feel normal; in four months, his medicine intake for colitis had come down to zero. He did have a relapse when he reintroduced dairy (bleeding when passing stool, low haemoglobin and high inflammatory markers). After that relapse, he swore he would not touch dairy products. He has also gained some weight, 6 kg, and now has a normal BMI.

The Case of the Epileptic Lady

Ms J. was twenty-three years old and had a history of epilepsy from the age of twelve (she was on medication for this). She'd been quite ill since childhood (tuberculosis when she was four years old and then typhoid). Fevers were frequent over the last decade too. Not unnaturally, she'd become depressed at twenty-two (and was being treated for it), and for the last three years, hadn't left her room or often, even her bed. She slept most of the day because of the medicines and was abusive at night; it was impossible for her to attend college. She was a very fussy eater as a child.

Most of her family and friends had given up on her; even the doctors were suggesting that she be tied up and taken to a rehab centre at a premier hospital in India.

Presenting Symptoms

- Epilepsy
- Breathlessness; poor eyesight
- Frequent stomach aches and a bad case of acne

Investigation revealed low haemoglobin, vitamin D and vitamin B12. Her celiac markers were negative. She hadn't been breastfed as a baby and had been given cow's milk right at the beginning. Her mother had suffered jaundice during her pregnancy.

I told her mother that she was suffering from a leaky gut because of wheat and it was worsened by medication. She changed her diet instantly. We eliminated inflammatory grains and dairy. Within a few weeks, there was a magical transformation. She felt better overall and normal sleep patterns were established. She'd had to leave her studies but her improved health made it possible for her to complete her education and begin working. The change completely transformed her life. She was down to only the epilepsy pill and off the cocktail of seven other drugs she was on.

The Case of the Arthritic Patient

Ms S. was not overweight (56 kg and a BMI of 23) but she suffered a lot of pain in her joints and was an emotional eater. She came in order to lose just a few kilos. She was on Folifrax for the arthritis but still complained of pain.

Presenting Symptoms

Rheumatoid arthritis, with severe joint pain, in spite of drug therapy.

Blood tests revealed her RA factor was 123, which is a high positive. Among other inflammatory markers, her calprotectin was 72, which should have been less than 50. Her haemoglobin was normal but ferritin levels were low. Lipoprotein A, which is a risk factor for developing heart disease, was high too, at 84.5.

When I told her that I was more interested in treating her arthritis, she said her doctor had told her she would have to be on lifelong medication for this autoimmune disorder. After I put her on a gluten-free, anti-inflammatory modified grain diet, her RA factor came down to 11 and then even to 8.8 in time. Other inflammatory markers also normalized. Lipoprotein is a marker that cannot be manipulated through treatment, but in those who go gluten-free, it comes down, and hers reached normal levels too.

She was pain-free, though, on a trip to Singapore, she had sushi with soya sauce—and the pain came right back. She removed it from her diet and felt better soon. When she approached menopause, she began having digestive issues. We then suggested she remove dairy and she was restored to her former health. Her quality of life was transformed and her pill burden was reduced to a fraction. On one of her visits, she became so emotional about her recovery that she bent down and touched my feet; a moment for me to cherish as a practitioner!

The Diabetic, Depressed Lady

Mrs B. came to us at the age of fifty-one. She had a weight issue; she weighed 87 kg and had a BMI of 36. She'd begun gaining weight after she had a baby (she was 49 kg earlier). Soon after, at thirty years, she developed depression and was put on antidepressants. She then proceeded to gain a kilo every year over the next twenty years and developed diabetes.

Presenting Symptoms

- Diabetes
- Depression
- Poor digestion, gastritis, low energy, poor appetite
- Knee pain

Investigation showed severe nutritional deficiencies of vitamin D, B12 and iron. She had fatty liver grade 2 and was losing proteins in her urine. Her CRP was a high 11.8, her HbA1C was 9.8 (despite diabetic medicines) and fasting sugar was 234. We modified the grains, gradually removed dairy and gave her a restorative diet. Probiotics and other supplements were added to build the gut, improve gut flora balance and address the deficiencies.

The results were transformational: by the end of the treatment, all her medications were removed, including supportive ones for the digestive issues. Within four months, she'd reached a weight of 74 kg and, without medicines, her HbA1C was 7.1. The antidepressants took longer to remove. She lost 15 kg, with a 10-kg loss in the first six months. And all this occurred while she was in the first phase of menopause, a time when such issues are usually aggravated. It's now been three years and she hasn't regained weight. Her diabetes was reversed and she is no longer depressed or on antidepressants. She's eternally grateful.

A Case of Reversing Infertility

A thirty-three-year-old educationist consulted us; she was morbidly obese (115 kg, BMI of 42) despite being a frugal eater. She had a history of childhood obesity. She'd gained a lot of weight also as a result of the fertility treatment.

Presenting Symptoms

- Recently detected as hypothyroid (was on a low dose of thyroid meds)
- Knee and shoulder pain, cracked feet, was on painkillers
- Could not conceive, despite many rounds of hormone treatment

Investigation showed her inflammatory markers were positive, though she was not nutritionally deficient. Her bloodwork showed that she was pre-diabetic. We removed the offending grains and gave her supplements to improve her gut health.

Interestingly, she lost hardly any weight (just 4 kg), but her aches and pains were all resolved. Most important, she conceived within six months. Her infertility issues had been reversed by dietary changes.

The Case of the 'Imbalanced' Businessman

Mr L., sixty-six, lived in South-east Asia, and had developed diabetes fifteen years before. He had a range of other issues as well, of which the biggest was ataxia, which signifies an inability to coordinate one's muscles when performing a voluntary movement; in his case, walking. It's not a disease in itself, but a sign of an underlying medical problem.

Presenting Symptoms

- Diabetes
- Reflux, candidiasis and low energy
- Hearing problems, fungus-related nail problems
- Ataxia, stiff shoulders, the beginning of arthritis

Investigation showed his anti-gliadin antibodies were positive, which revealed a gluten sensitivity. His celiac markers were negative. He had normal Hb levels but vitamin D, B12 and magnesium levels were low and his CRP was elevated.

But soon after he was put on a gluten- and dairy-free diet, many of the issues were resolved. He wasn't closely monitored because he lived overseas and consulted infrequently but his blood sugar came down to normal and the ataxia improved significantly. His gait became more balanced and coordinated.

A Placental Crossover Case

This sixteen-year-old boy had been very underweight at birth and seemed too small for his age. He'd always had digestive issues but his family had not realized that this was a problem.

Presenting Symptoms

- Needed to go to the loo as soon as he ate
- Growth seemed poor and he had a hunchback
- Low energy

Scans showed that one of his kidneys had not developed and bloodwork revealed high haemoglobin (17.7) calcium levels and low ferritin. Liver enzymes were abnormal and levels of bilirubin, antibodies for thyroid and TSH levels were high. The celiac markers were negative.

As soon as he was put on a gluten-free diet, his digestive issues began to resolve. His energy levels and confidence improved dramatically and he began walking straighter. Thyroid levels came down to normal.

Although there are no tests to confirm this, from the fact that his mother was gluten-intolerant, one can hypothesize that antibodies had crossed over from the placenta and harmed the growth of the infant, attacking the development of the liver, kidneys, the gut and the thyroid. His sister too had PCOD, thyroid issues and a case of OCD. The child has embraced the modified diet to a T. He feels much better, confident, is straight-backed and the reports are all normal.

The Fantastic Case of the Golfer Child

Vitamin D is called the sunshine vitamin and is synthesized in the body during exposure to the sun. In the case of this young lad, his father was a caddy and he too had played golf all his life, so he got plenty of sun exposure. He came in for a consultation in 2015, aged 11, because he seemed stuck at four feet ten and he was just 36 kg.

Presenting Symptoms

Hadn't gained any height for two years.

Blood tests showed his haemoglobin was 14.3 but his ferritin was low and so was his Vitamin D, even though he got loads of sunshine every day. He came from an underprivileged background so we did not suggest major sensitivity tests; we simply empirically applied grain science, eliminated inflammatory grains and added a multivitamin supplement to correct the nutritional deficiencies.

The results were dramatic: he got a height spurt, gaining 1.5 inches in four months and 4.5 inches over the year. His game also improved with better hand-eye coordination and he began winning international championships. He's now sixteen years old and is five feet eight, the tallest in his family. He's also an international-level golfer in his age category and is a TED Talks speaker. This was a case that showed clearly that if gut flora are imbalanced, malabsorption is sure to kick in.

(**Note:** this is an observational study; we didn't have enough serology to document sensitivity, but the results were dramatic.)

The Case of the Constantly Tired Lady

The wife of a senior police official with an export business of her own came with complaints of low energy and high body fat. She was already perimenopausal at the age of forty-two. Her BMI was not high (24), but she was slightly overweight.

Presenting Symptoms

- Felt as if she had the energy of an elderly person
- Recent hair fall
- Polyp recently removed from her uterus because of heavy bleeding

Her bloodwork showed low iron and ferritin levels. She was already taking a vitamin D supplement. She also had elevated thyroid antibodies. Her celiac markers were negative. We modified her grains, corrected her nutritional deficiencies and built up her gut flora; she also decided to go vegan on her own.

Within weeks, she began losing weight (she lost 6 kg) and her BMI came down to 21. Her skin was soon glowing, and she reported feeling clear in the head and all perked up. Her menses were also more regulated. She said, 'At the age of forty-six, by changing your food, you can change your life, your mood and look like a happy child.'

The Lady Who Could Hardly Walk

Mrs J., an architect, fifty-nine years old, was hardly able to walk on her own when she came to us. She needed someone to support her; she'd been asked to undergo knee surgery. She was overweight (115 kg, five feet five), with a BMI of 48. She'd had a hysterectomy eleven years earlier; then her ovaries were removed and she began gaining weight. She was also on medication for high blood pressure and diabetes.

Presenting Symptoms

- Adult acne since the age of forty-three, hair fall
- High blood pressure
- Diabetes
- Incontinence
- Varicose veins

Bloodwork showed elevated CRP (11) and blood sugar levels, normal Hb but low vitamin D. Inflammatory grains were removed from her diet and within the first weight loss of just 2 kg, she found herself able to walk without support. Within a month, she was so comfortable that she began taking on new work projects.

Over a period of eighteen months, she lost a staggering 37 kg, to reach 77 kg. Her diabetes medication was reduced and then stopped. For four years, she also avoided knee surgery. She finally had the knee operation but continues to maintain her diet and weight loss regimen.

The Lady with Hypoglycemia

Ms H., just thirty-four, came five years ago with severe digestive issues. She was obese (92 kg) and her blood sugar levels would plummet; when she ate anything sweet, she would begin shivering and have to rush to the loo. She was also on medication for her thyroid.

Presenting Symptoms

- High blood pressure, fatty liver grade 2, acne, hair fall, migraine and vertigo
- Severe reactive hypoglycemia
- Acid reflux, sleep apnea
- Heavy bleeding in menses

Her tests showed high creatinine levels, low haemoglobin (11.1), an elevated CRP (9.9) and her blood sugar was over 100. Her ferritin levels were very low (19). The celiac markers were negative. We modified her diet, removing inflammatory grains but working with her took time as she didn't keep to the diet; she would contaminate it by eating foods that contained gluten. Part of the reason was that she had several doctors in her family, who would question whether diet could help resolve any of her issues.

But she began to lose weight (she's now 69 kg). She's committed to the dietary change, having seen the benefit. Her blood markers have all normalized and the hypoglycemia has resolved. In fact, she had an eight-year-old child who had severe anxiety, tics, involuntary jerking and weakness. After adopting a gluten-free and dairy-free diet, he's responding well to the change. Most of his issues are resolved.

The Case of a Family Intolerance

Mrs S. came in nine years ago; she was fifty-six years old then and an active golfer. She wanted to lose weight. She had some pain issues and occasional acidity.

Presenting Symptoms

- Knee and lower back pain
- Fatigue, irritability, hair fall, brittle nails
- Occasional acid reflux

On screening, her CRP and anti-gliadin levels were high. But what was much more interesting was that she turned out to be a case of full-blown celiac disease, though atypical, with most of her symptoms outside the gut. She naturally had to go off gluten for life—but because she was celiac-positive, her grandchildren, who were plump and lethargic, also came in for testing.

On screening, both turned out to be intolerant to gluten and one was celiac-positive. Her son also was gluten-intolerant. The whole family is now responding well to a gluten-free diet. This is a case where because of one person in the family, the food triggers for the entire family were discovered. The learning is clear that screening of first-degree relatives is essential, regardless of symptoms.

A Case of Celiac-Caused Palsy

Ms K., aged thirty-two, was just shy of being obese (87 kg at five feet five). She had a range of skin issues including psoriasis and facial paralysis called Bell's Palsy. She was on medicines for hypertension and on anti-anxiety pills, which made her sleep a lot. She wasn't able to lose weight. Both her parents were diabetic; her father had died of lung cancer and her mother suffered from depression.

Presenting Symptoms

- Psoriasis
- Bell's Palsy
- Hypertension since the age of twenty-four

Investigation showed several deficiencies (low vitamin D and B12), critically high uric acid, elevated thyroid antibodies and an abnormal lipid profile. The anti-gliadin antibodies were also high and scanning showed inflammation in the small intestine, so I suggested a biopsy, which was clear.

But it was her celiac marker (first at 144 and then 226 in a repeat test, when normal is under 20) that showed she had full-blown celiac disease. She responded very well to the complete elimination of gluten from her diet, lost 10 kg in six months and resolved most other issues, including the anxiety.

The Case of the Returning Dermatitis

A super-fit forty-year-old lady came in with some skin issues and very minor digestive ones. She was five feet six and weighed 48 kg, with a BMI of 19. The sister of a homoeopath, she'd consulted many doctors over the last three to four years for the black patches on her neck. Medically, she was only on a few vitamin supplements.

Presenting Symptoms

- Seborrheic dermatitis since 2016, with itchiness and patches on the neck and white flakes on the eyelashes
- Acidity for six to seven years

Her bloodwork showed a magnesium, vitamin D and vitamin B12 deficiency. Two months into a modification of her diet and elimination of inflammatory grains, her skin issues were completely resolved. However, she returned after a year to report that the patches were coming back—this, while she was strictly gluten-free.

That seemed odd, as she had immediately responded well to a gluten-free diet, so I did a little detective work. I asked her what atta she was consuming. We discovered that though the atta was indeed gluten-free, it was a different variety, though from the same brand that she had been using. This one contained soya, which had caused a cross-reaction. She changed to one without both gluten and soya and was sorted. The power of dietary change was obvious. The issue of cross-reactivity was once again reinforced.

The Boy Who Never Went to School

This thirteen-year-old child had never really gone to school; his attention-deficit disorder was so severe that he simply couldn't sit in class. He was also obese, at 102 kg, and just over five feet seven. Bespectacled, lazy and passive, he had zero motivation to make any changes to his lifestyle. He ate constantly and in large portions; he would regularly eat five to six chapatis in a meal.

Presenting Symptoms

- Severe attention-deficit disorder (ADD) and on medication for it
- Obesity

On investigation, we found very low levels of vitamin D (just 13.6), B12 (188) and ferritin. His celiac markers were negative, but the anti-gliadin antibodies were borderline positive, suggesting a non-celiac wheat sensitivity. His mother, who had accompanied her son and wanted to achieve weight loss, also tested positive for anti-gliadin antibodies. Her celiac markers too were negative. This reinforces the fact that often, such sensitivities run in families.

We eliminated gluten and cross-reactive grains from his diet. It took him several months to embrace a gluten-free lifestyle, but once he did, he began to lose weight. After three months, I happened to ask his mother how he was doing academically. She said he'd sat for an exam for the first time in his life. She hadn't reported the fact that he was sitting and studying for hours, because they hadn't correlated this change with the diet. He soon went on to write his own board exams and secured 84 per cent. Unreal!

After eight to ten years, he continues to remain diligent about dietary compliance. He now looks like a model and has gained the confidence to be a public speaker. He spoke in our Celiac Society meeting and said he'd never imagined speaking in public. Both he and his mother welled up. A life transformed!

The Case of the Rumbling Stomach

Mr B., a south Indian businessman, the son of a legendary actor and dancer from the South, forty-five years old, came with very severe borborygmi (sounds from the stomach). He felt uneasy in the pit of his stomach whenever he ate. He had been prescribed antacids but they hadn't helped. He was on vitamin supplements and Ayurvedic preparations but the discomfort persisted. He was slim, with a BMI of 20, and was a teetotaler.

Presenting Symptoms

- Severe rumbling after a meal
- Gastroesophageal reflux disease (GERD) and heartburn

He was well-connected, so there had been many kinds of investigations, but no cause for the problem had been identified. His bloodwork revealed a deficiency of vitamin D, low levels of vitamin B12, hypothyroid and fatty liver grade 1. His tTG marker (for celiac disease) was negative.

Certain he was still gluten-intolerant, we put him on a modified grain diet. He began responding positively to the elimination within days. The acid reflux resolved and the irritating and embarrassing sounds from the stomach began to die down. He now follows the modified grain diet and has resumed normal work, which he couldn't because of the embarrassing rumbling sounds, until now.

The Case of the Too-Thin Man

Mr S., sixty-five, came with a history of digestive issues and low immunity. He would fall sick easily. He had a low BMI of 18 and was underweight, at just 56 kg. Despite being too thin and the fact that he was very careful about his diet, he was borderline diabetic. He was also on antidepressant medicines for a few months.

Presenting Symptoms

- Had a stroke because of low sodium
- Underactive thyroid
- Was often ill, got frequent sore throats

His haemoglobin was quite low (8–9), but the vitamin B12 levels were high; this is usually a picture that accompanies chronic inflammation. Our analysis was that this was a case of malabsorption. I told him to go gluten-free, in order to take care of his inability to gain weight and to help with his recent depression. He followed the diet strictly and came up to 62 kg, didn't get a sore throat and moved off the antidepressants in just a few months. A changed life!

First-Person Accounts

The Case of the Non-Expectant Mother

'Soon after I got married, my mother-in-law began asking me if I was pregnant. I was putting on weight and was often nauseous after a meal. But it soon turned out to be just bloating. Even when I was actually expecting a baby, I was absolutely miserable with my inability to digest what I was eating. I continued to eat everything. Some years later, I had such severe rage issues that if someone edged me out of my lane, I would want to stop and start screaming at the offender.

'I didn't know until many years later, when I came to the clinic, that it was the wheat-related items in my diet that I was so severely allergic to. Since knowing my sensitivity to gluten and eliminating it from my diet (*her celiac markers were tested several times and were negative*), I now know what was troubling me so much earlier. I feel so much better, more in control of myself and over my anger issues.'

Life-Changing Plan

'I went to Dr Ishi Khosla with the most basic problem—weight gain. With a move to a new city and the challenges that came with it, indulging in food became a comfort, and I simply hadn't realized how much weight I was slowly putting on. That's the thing with weight; it is a few grams up today and a few more the next day, until you actually look back and realize that those few grams have added up to rather a lot of kilos.

'There is also a back story to this weight gain, which is why there was some panic upon the harsh realization of how much. I had been operated upon for a gall bladder cyst removal when I was sixteen and since then my body didn't like food as much as I did. And although we got rid of the problem with the operation, the pain never quite went away.

'I had also developed a thyroid issue when I was pretty young and almost all my family members have a problem with obesity. So, when I added up all of this, I needed to find a solution, a better way of indulging in food and yet make sure that whatever I ate did not harm me in any way. At the same time, I was also going through menopause, which came with its own set of problems.

'Dr Ishi Khosla's diet plan has helped me maintain my love for food and at the same time ensured that all that I eat helps strengthen my system internally, rather than cause more trouble. The plan was much more about nutrition than actual "dieting". The first two months were a little difficult because there was a lot to think about in terms of what was good and what was not; it was also about rewiring one's brain to look at food from a very holistic angle. And once it was in place, the plan was about sincerity. And it has paid off—in spades!'

A Case of Severe Endometriosis

'I came in 2018 when I was suffering from severe pain in my uterus. For about fifteen days in a month, I was in a lot of pain and during the first, second and third days of my menses, I had to be on a drip. Living in a joint family, outings and family functions were planned around my period dates. My gynaecologist told me that I had endometriosis of the third grade and that I had to be put on hormonal treatments. I did begin taking the medication, but there were many side effects; I was gaining weight and my hair started falling as well.

Fortunately, my brother-in-law had consulted with the clinic for his gut-related issues, so he directed me here.

'Within three months of moving to a gluten-free diet, I got my results. My periods became painless, almost like magic. My whole month was pain-free and I was so happy—that it was life-changing for me. Also, during this time, my weight dropped from 67 to 60 kg. Earlier, the endometriosis was so high that I had had trouble conceiving; this happened during my treatment at the clinic.'

The Strange Case of the Paper-Eater

'Until two months ago, I was simply fed up. Just twenty-seven years old, I had been suffering for the last fourteen years from what anyone would imagine was a weird habit, that of eating paper. I discovered that there was actually a clinical term for it, PICA (a psychological disorder in which there is an appetite for substances that do not have nutritive value).

'As a professionally qualified woman, I simply couldn't understand why I couldn't kick this habit. I had visited several different doctors, who did symptomatic treatment but never reached the root cause of my problem. When it persisted, I tried to keep the topic of having kids in abeyance in chats with my husband, as I was fearful of the harmful effects my habit might have on my yet-to-be-born kids.

'But then, after we had an intense fight about my paper-eating, my husband took it upon himself to find a solution, He researched it extensively, found a case history similar to mine and read up on the successful treatment. Given that this was a doctor abroad, we thought of trying to find a similar specialist in India.

'After asking around, I came across Ms Ishi through a friend who recommended her; we learnt that she was one of the eminent professionals regarding celiac disease. We approached Ms Ishi, who was instantly able to confirm my symptoms of low iron and other nutrients, coupled with the paper-eating, as being linked to celiac disease. Her way of conversation and patient hearing put me at ease and gave me confidence in my ability to kick this persistent habit. The great thing is that she has been able to just look at my food diary and suggest tweaks in case of any gastric or other issues.

'For the first time in thirteen years, I am a happy person. Paper-eating, hopefully, is a thing of the past.'

Notes: Decoding the Figures

- BMI measure is kg/m2; the normal range is 18.5–24.9.
- Waist circumference should be less than 31.5 inches for women and less than 35.5 inches for men.
- Haemoglobin for women should be over 12 to 15.5 gm/dL; for men between 13.5 and 17.5 gm/dL.
- Fasting blood sugar should be under 100 mg/dL, 100–125 is considered prediabetes; more than that is diabetic; HbA1C or three-month average should be between 4 and 5.6 per cent.
- Ferritin levels range between 12 and 300 ng/mL for men and between 12 and 150 ng/mL for women.
- Vitamin D levels of under 20 ng/mL are considered deficient; between 40 and 60 ng/mL are ideal.
- Vitamin B12: Under 200 pg/mL is borderline deficient; between 200 and 950 pg/mL is normal.
- CRP is measured in milligrams per litre. Normal levels are usually below 3.0 mg/L.
- Tests for celiac disease are tissue transglutaminase antibodies (tTG-IgA) tests; a negative result means that the person does not have celiac disease.
- People with non-celiac gluten sensitivity (NCGS) either have symptoms similar to celiac disease or present a wide range of atypical symptoms, most of which resolve when gluten is removed from their diet. There is no specific blood test for NCGS; one needs to first rule out celiac disease, then do a food intolerance test, which includes gluten and other

common allergens, such as milk, eggs and nuts. As can be seen from many of the cases, if a patient's finances do not support expensive testing, a simple elimination process and food challenge can reveal a great deal to the diet detective.

From the Author's Desk

This book has been a culmination of my learnings over twenty-five years of clinical experience. I have had the privilege of meeting each and every client personally (they are referred to as patients since I started in a hospital and worked there for seven years) and understanding their singular needs and individual dietary triggers. The richness of these interactions is something I understood much later; as much as I had to guide them on to the road to health, I learnt something—and often, many things—from each of them and their cases.

As the clients and I worked together to understand and resolve their health issues, I too grew as a professional—due in no small measure to the information provided from their serological testing and their verbal feedback. Personal and family medical histories are a great way to contour the edges of a client's issues and present health conditions. Detailed interaction on their response to medicines, supplements and to the diet modifications helps to begin filling in the picture. The bloodwork helps to scientifically confirm the diagnosis. Their ability to stick to the dietary changes in the long term and the social, cultural and psychological impact on their eating behaviour, all work together to form the full picture. If I compiled all the details, each case could become an individual research paper in itself!

Over the decades, however, patterns emerged in diagnosis, testing and diet planning. Even stray pieces of evidence became clear clues to the detection of a particular intolerance or deficiency.

In this book, I have poured the distilled knowledge of the impact of the four Gs—the Gut, our Girth, food sensitivities to Gluten and other allergens, and the effect of Glucose and similar addictive foods—on all our chronic health conditions. Most important, the fact that this influence is through their combined effect on eating behaviour and vice versa.

I firmly believe that everyone—even the man on the street—*knows* what to eat and what not to. A person may have issues in getting sufficient, or safe, food. People in rural areas have access to the right food by default and therefore have relatively less exposure to unhealthy food. There is a global 'ill health epidemic', caused by modern, stressful lifestyles as well as polluted air, water and soil that adversely affect the food we eat. The problem may be complex, but the solution is simple: safe, sufficient and sustainable food systems.

The urban educated people understand the difference between good food and bad food—but seem unable to stick to the right path. The reasons for the tilt towards unhealthy eating patterns are clear: from birth to adulthood, genetics, the mother's diet during pregnancy, her mental health, all these notes play out like a symphony, defining Us—inside out!

Yet, people are often unaware of whether there is an incipient health problem lurking in their future, at what age, with what intensity and if they can buy themselves an insurance policy against it.

They don't realize that they CAN!

What I want to tell my readers in this book is that the manifestation of health issues is intricately linked to the impact of dietary and environmental factors on our genes and on our eating behaviour. But this is a dynamic process and, just as the gene for height can exist in us, poor diet and lack of exercise will adversely affect how much we actually grow; the expression of any genetic predisposition to ill health too can be countered by altered diets and lifestyles.

This knowledge is humbling but true: all of us can change both our present and future health. For the practitioner, the gratification that comes from simply being able to examine the evidentiary clues and arrive at a life-changing diagnosis—and often reverse chronic disorders and diseases successfully—is an absolutely exhilarating experience.

But if the experience is empowering for the practitioner, for the patient it can be transformational. Yes, the road may be somewhat bumpy to begin with, but with support and hand-holding, the rewards are there for the taking. And the complete makeover—in self-confidence, overall well-being and being healthy—is a delight. Once that happens, it motivates almost every one of my clients to embrace the altered lifestyle and make it their own.

I call it the DIET Dividend. It represents a return to youthful energy and the joy of reclaimed health.

My own learnings through this experience are simple and clear:

- All of us want to live healthy;
- We usually know what is right for us, but the knowledge is not in focus;
- This is why it's difficult for us to stay on the path;
- When we get the insights from the science of the four Gs and their interplay, we can join the dots and understand the connections;
- And then be poised to modify eating behaviour and lifestyle in a permanent manner.
- We are not only what we eat, but what we digest—and what we DON'T eat!
- Our bodies are forgiving and capable of healing. It's NEVER too late!

I would like to convey my heartfelt thanks to all those who have helped shape my career and learnings. In this, the first people I want to thank are my patients; they trusted me with their health and they had faith in me.

An event that accelerated my learning curve was Dr Tom O'Bryan's Gluten E-Summit. It helped me validate my practice and introduced me to a galaxy of globally-respected professionals who were on the same page as I was. These included Dr Marsh, Dr Alessio Fasano, Dr Mark Hyman, Dr Natasha Campbell, Dr Rodney Ford, and the father of autoimmunity, Dr Yehuda Shoenfeld. It was so exciting to hear them and read their scientific publications.

For me, this was a time when I knew what I was doing on the dietary front was correct but my medical colleagues were dismissive and not convinced. The whole concept of the existence of wheat sensitivity without celiac disease was just not acceptable. Patients too were sceptical, since their physicians discouraged them from using dietary change to get on the path to health. I'm truly indebted to Dr Tom for putting together the e-summit and getting like-minded professionals on the same platform.

Among those whom I'd like to thank for this book is Vidhu Khanna, who helped me put this manuscript together. I shared all my writings and case studies with her and she offered to help me give it shape. I would also like to thank Divya Parashar for her informed and valuable suggestions on the book.

Others who have been invaluable include all my office colleagues, especially Shivani Sharma, who spent many hours combing through case files and collating information.

None of this work would have been possible without the support provided by my family: I want to thank them for being the pillars of my life. They have supported me physically and emotionally. Their patience has been the only way I could complete this book.

Last, but definitely not least, I'd like to thank my publishers, who reposed faith in my work and who have helped publish my previous books as well.

—Ishi Khosla

Notes

Chapter I: The Gut Matters

1 R.K. Singh, H.W. Chang, D. Yan et al. 'Influence of Diet on the Gut Microbiome and Implications for Human Health', *J. Transl. Med.* 15, 73 (2017). https://doi.org/10.1186/s12967-017-1175-y
2 National Family Health Survey-4.
3 World Cancer Report, 2020.
4 CDC, 2018.
5 Alessio Fasano, PMC, F. 1000 Research, January 2020.

Chapter II: The 4-G Connectivity

1 *Journal of American Medical Association*, 2016.

Chapter III: Why Wheat-Related Disorders Are on the Rise

1 Makharia, 2011.
2 BMC, 2019.

3 Sapone et al., 2012; Quinn et al., 1999; Carneval et al., 2014; Valerii et al. 2015.

4 R. Raman, 2017; F. Truzzi, 2022; *International Journal of Molecular Sciences*, 27113425

5 J. Grovers, *Frontiers of Immunology*, 2019.

6 MDP/Journals, Foods 2022, Vol. 11, Issue 11.

7 M. de Lorgeril, and P. Salen, 2014.

8 *Journal of Cereal Science*, January 2018; Careggi University Hospital, Florence, 2013.

9 BioMed Central, December 2020.

10 www.jvs.org.uk

11 Bikaner University study, 2013.

12 Mahmoud Kandeel, Wael El-Deeb, PMC Bioinorganic Chemistry, April 2022.

13 R.P. Agarwal et al., *Diabetes Research and Clinical Practice*, Volume 68, Issue 2, p. 0176–77, 1 May 2005.

14 Joanna K. Winstone, et al., *Journal of Neuroinflammation*, 193, 2022.

Chapter IV: Wheat and Weight

1 Carlo Catassi, *Annals of Medicine*, 2010.

Chapter V: Glucose: The Dark Side

1 Jamie C. Honohan, '13, Rebecca H. Markson, '13, Lauren Cameron, '14.

2 Ages, March 2022.

Chapter VI: Girth: Figure It Out

1 Bodil Ohlsson, Marju Orho-Melander and Peter M. Nilsson, PMC, *International Journal of Molecular Science*, March 2017.

2 Christopher Wanjek, 'Food at Work: Work Place Solution for Malnutrition, Obesity and Chronic Disease', International Labour Organization, 2005.

Chapter VII: The P Factors: Thirty-Five Leads to a Leaky Gut

1 Timothy and Emma, MDPI, *Nutrients* 2019, 11 (10), 2364.

2 Dept. of Animal and Dairy Sciences, April 2022.

3 Gibson and Roverford, *J. Nutrition*, June 1995.

4 *Annu. Rev. Food Science Technology*, National Library of Medicine, 2011.

5 Jaime Ramirez, Francisco Guarner, 'Frontiers in Cellular and Infection Microbiology', October 2020.

6 Sofia et al.

7 K. Lu and Ryan Phillip, *Environmental Health Perspectives* 122; 284–291, 2014.

8 Philipp Schwabl et al., *Ann. Internal Medicine*, National Library of Medicine, 2019.

9 Hermosa Study, UC Berkeley.

10 *Journal of Nature Communications*, Belgium 2019.

11 Nutrients PMC, May 2019.

12 B. Dorelli, F. Gallè, C. De Vito, G. Duranti, Nutrients, 31 May 2021.

13 Blackhead et al., 2015; Collado et al., 2012.

Chapter VIII: Food for Thought

1 PMC Nature Reviews, *Neuroscience* 02; Fernando Gomes 2008.
2 Michael D. Gershon, Columbia University.
3 Bercik et al., 2014.
4 B. Baspinar, *The Eurasian Journal of Medicine*, 2020.

Chapter XI: The Third P

1 National Institute of Health, 2001.
2 PLOS ONE, October 2019.
3 M. Nedergaord, *Science Translational Medicine*, 2013.

Chapter XII: Immunity: A Formidable Weapon

1 Chuen Wen Tan, Liam Pock Ho et al., 'A Cohort Study to Evaluate the Effect of Combination Vitamin D, Magnesium and Vitamin B12 (DMB) on Progression to Severe Outcome in Older COVID-19 patients', medRxiv, 2 June 2020, https://www.medrxiv.org/content/10.1101/2020.06.01.20112334v1
2 Harvard T.H. Chan School of Public Health, the Nutrition Source.
3 *Journal of Inorganic Biochemistry*, Volume 228, March 2022, 111691.
4 *European Journal of Pharmacology*, Elsevier, 2020.
5 *Time*, July 2020.
6 Obesity, Research & Clinical Practices, 2021.

7 L. Jimenez, 'Death by COVID-19', 2021, cited by 17—The Severe Acute Respiratory Syndrome Coronavirus.
8 Yi Huang, Yao Lu, PMC Elsevier Public Health Emergency Collection, September 2020.